Dermatology at a Glance

Mahbub M.U. Chowdhury

MBChB, FRCP
Consultant Dermatologist
The Welsh Institute of Dermatology
University Hospital of Wales
Cardiff, UK

Ruwani P. Katugampola

BM, MRCP, MD (Cardiff)
Consultant Dermatologist
The Welsh Institute of Dermatology
University Hospital of Wales
Cardiff, UK

Andrew Y. Finlay

CBE, MBBS, FRCP (London), FRCP (Glasgow)
Professor of Dermatology
Department of Dermatology and Wound Healing
Cardiff University School of Medicine
Cardiff, UK

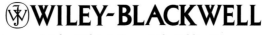
WILEY-BLACKWELL

A John Wiley & Sons, Ltd., Publication

This edition first published 2013 © 2013 by John Wiley & Sons, Ltd

Wiley-Blackwell is an imprint of John Wiley & Sons, formed by the merger of Wiley's global Scientific, Technical and Medical business with Blackwell Publishing.

Registered office: John Wiley & Sons, Ltd, The Atrium, Southern Gate, Chichester, West Sussex, PO19 8SQ, UK

Editorial offices: 9600 Garsington Road, Oxford, OX4 2DQ, UK
The Atrium, Southern Gate, Chichester, West Sussex, PO19 8SQ, UK
111 River Street, Hoboken, NJ 07030-5774, USA

For details of our global editorial offices, for customer services and for information about how to apply for permission to reuse the copyright material in this book please see our website at www.wiley.com/wiley-blackwell.

Library of Congress Cataloging-in-Publication Data
Chowdhury, Mahbub M. U.
  Dermatology at a glance / Mahbub M.U. Chowdhury, Ruwani P. Katugampola,
Andrew Y. Finlay.
    p. cm.
  Includes bibliographical references and index.
  ISBN 978-0-470-65673-0 (pbk. : alk. paper) 1. Dermatology. 2. Skin–Diseases.
I. Katugampola, Ruwani
P. II. Finlay, Andrew Y. III. Title.
  RL74.C46 2013
  616.5–dc23
                          2012007647

A catalogue record for this book is available from the British Library.

Wiley also publishes its books in a variety of electronic formats. Some content that appears in print may not be available in electronic books.

Cover design: Andy Meaden

Set in 9/11.5 pt Times by Toppan Best-set Premedia Limited
Printed and bound in Malaysia by Vivar Printing Sdn Bhd

1 2013

Contents

Companion website

A companion website is available at:

www.ataglanceseries.com/dermatology

featuring:
- Summary revision notes
- Interactive case studies
- Downloadable figures from the book
- Further reading list

Preface

This book is especially designed for medical students, general practitioners and nurses with a special interest in dermatology. You will find all the facts to help you pass dermatology undergraduate exams. It is also a great starting point when studying for higher exams such as the MRCP or MRCGP. It gives you the basics in clear understandable language and then builds on them.

All you need to know about each topic is presented on one open spread. This attractive double page layout is an ideal format for studying and revising. This book uses all the experience that has made the 'At a Glance' series highly successful. Clear original diagrams and tables make complex subjects simple and there are over 300 clinical photographs. We have highlighted any key points and specific clinical warnings across the book. There is a Best of the Web section to guide your online dermatology searches.

Dermatology at a Glance is written by three experts in clinical dermatology, who have special expertise in skin allergy, paediatric dermatology, medical dermatology and quality of life. They are all based in the Cardiff Dermatology Department, which is known internationally as a world leader in dermatology education (www. dermatology.org.uk).

Clinical dermatology is a fascinating subject. We hope that reading this book will help you become as enthusiastic as we are about the largest organ in the body, the skin, and its clinical challenges.

Mahbub M.U. Chowdhury
Ruwani P. Katugampola
Andrew Y. Finlay
Cardiff

About the authors

Mahbub M.U. Chowdhury MBChB, FRCP
Dr Chowdhury is Treasurer of the British Society for Cutaneous Allergy and Medical Secretary for the UK Dermatology Specialty Exam Board. He is an international expert in skin allergy and has over 70 published articles and book chapters and has co-edited two other textbooks. He has over 15 years' experience in dermatology teaching for medical students and was Chairman for Dermatology registrar training in Wales. His research interests include latex allergy, occupational dermatology and contact dermatitis.

Ruwani P. Katugampola BM, MRCP, MD (Cardiff)
Dr Katugampola has a special interest in Paediatric Dermatology and has over 20 published papers and book chapters. She is involved in dermatology education by teaching and examining medical students and postgraduate doctors. Her research interests include rare congenital cutaneous porphyrias and the development of a national clinical service for these individuals.

Andrew Y. Finlay CBE, MBBS, FRCP (London), FRCP (Glasgow)
Professor Andrew Finlay was previously Head of the Academic Dermatology Department at Cardiff University. He has been involved in dermatology education for over 30 years, and created the highly successful distance-learning international Diploma in Practical Dermatology for GPs. His research has focused on developing ways to measure the impact that skin disease has on people's lives and on their families: questionnaires developed by his team are now used routinely across the world.

Foreword

When I was a medical student, I craved for short textbooks that would quickly give me an overview of the important things to learn in a topic such as dermatology, so that I could see the wood for the trees and get a sense of the whole rather than the details. And if that book also had lots of summary tables, key points and illustrations, I was in heaven. Thankfully, the medical students of today, and also others such as general practitioners and nurses who want a succinct overview of the important bits of dermatology, are blessed with this book *Dermatology at a Glance* by Chowdhury, Katugampola and Finlay. Writing succinctly is not easy, and trying to capture each topic on a double-paged spread like the other *At a Glance* series is challenging, yet the authors have succeeded in getting the right balance of detail, evidence and patient perspectives into this practical and useful book. It is also fun to read, especially with the quiz at the end. The authors have put a lot of thought into the book structure, and as well as the traditional topic-based layout including areas such as melanoma skin cancer, fungal infections and systemic disease, they have included sections such as 'the red face' or 'the elderly skin', or a 'child with a rash', because that is how people present in the real world. Written by a very experienced team who have delivered dermatology teaching for many years, the book is a masterpiece of entry level reading in dermatology. I commend it to all who are interested in finding out more about the skin in health and disease.

Hywel C. Williams MSc, PhD, FRCP
Professor of Dermato-Epidemiology and Director of the Centre of Evidence-Based Dermatology, University of Nottingham and Nottingham University Hospitals NHS Trust, Queen's Medical Centre, Nottingham, UK

Acknowledgements

We wish to thank and acknowledge the following for their input during the preparation of this book: our patients for having given signed permission for their clinical images to be published and our consultant colleagues for the use of clinical images of their patients including Dr Mazin Alfaham, Professor Alex Anstey, Dr Phil Atkins, Dr J. Davies, Dr Maria Gonzalez, Professor Keith Harding, Dr Peter Holt, Dr Manju Kalavala, Professor Mike Lewis, Dr Colin Long, Dr Andrew Morris, Dr Richard Motley, Dr Julian Nash, Dr Girish Patel, Professor Vincent Piguet, Dr Hamsaraj Shetty, Dr Graham Shortland, Dr David Tuthill, and Mr Patrick Watts. We would like to thank Dr Kenneth May for preparing the histology illustrations and Miss Fiona Ruge for the direct immunofluorescence images. We would like to thank all recent surgical fellows and specialist registrars who have organised specific photographs used in this book.

We would especially like to thank the clinical photographers of the Media Resources Centre, University Hospital of Wales, Cardiff for taking all of the clinical images and the Cardiff and Vale University Local Health Board, the copyright owner of all of the clinical images in this book, for permission to reproduce these images. We wish to thank the British Association of Dermatologists for permission to reproduce the photograph of Dr John Pringle. We also thank Mosby Elsevier for permission to reproduce figures from Chapter 12, Surgical Techniques (Dr P.J.A. Holt) In: A.Y. Finlay, M.M.U. Chowdhury (eds). *Specialist Training in Dermatology*, Edinburgh 2007, pp. 221, 224, 234, 240.

We would also like to thank our dedicated nursing staff in the Dermatology Day Treatment unit, University Hospital of Wales, Cardiff, for organising photographs of practical treatments and phototherapy.

We would like to thank Mrs Emma Williams for her excellent secretarial assistance, Dr Rachel Abbott, Sister Beverly Gambles, Sister Sue Parkes and Dr Dev Shah for their help with obtaining specific photographs and Dr John Ingram for reading the manuscript and making helpful suggestions. Dr Andrew Morris also kindly authorised administrative support.

Karen Moore provided excellent editorial support throughout the preparation of this book and we would like to thank her colleagues and the artist for the superb artwork.

We would like to thank all of our medical students who have inspired us to write this book for future generations of doctors.

Last, but not least, we wish to thank our families for their unfailing patience and support during the preparation of this book.

Conflict of interests

AYF is joint copyright owner of the DLQI, CDLQI and FDLQI: Cardiff University gains income from their use. AYF is a paid member of the Global Alliance to Improve Outcomes in Acne (funded by Galderma) and he has been a paid member of advisory boards to pharmaceutical companies who market biologics for psoriasis. AYF is chair of the UK Dermatology Clinical Trials Network Executive Group. MMC has been a paid consultant on advisory boards for Basilea.

List of abbreviations

ABPI	ankle brachial pressure index
ACD	allergic contact dermatitis
AD	atopic dermatitis
AIDS	acquired immunodeficiency syndrome
AIP	acute intermittent porphyria
AJCC	American Joint Committee on Cancer
ANA	antinuclear antibody
ANCA	anti-neutrophil cytoplasmic antibody
APC	antigen presenting cell
BAD	British Association of Dermatologists
BCC	basal cell carcinoma
BM	basement membrane
CDC	Centers for Disease Control and Prevention
CEP	congenital erythropoietic porphyria
CRP	C-reactive protein
CTCL	cutaneous T-cell lymphoma
DLE	discoid lupus erythematosus
DLQI	dermatology life quality index
DVT	deep vein thrombosis
EB	epidermolysis bullosa
ECG	electrocardiogram
EPP	erythropoietic protoporphyria
ESR	erythrocyte sedimentation rate
FBC	full blood count
FTU	finger tip unit
GvHD	graft versus host disease
HAART	highly active anti-retroviral treatment
HHV	human herpes virus
HIV	human immunodeficiency virus
HPV	human papilloma virus
HSV	herpes simplex virus
ICD	irritant contact dermatitis
Ig	immunoglobulin
IL	interleukin
IMF	immunofluorescence
IRIS	immune reconstitution inflammatory syndrome
KA	keratoacanthoma
KS	Kaposi's sarcoma
LASER	light amplification by stimulated emission of radiation
LP	lichen planus
LS	lichen sclerosus
MHC	major histocompatibility complex
MM	malignant melanoma
MMR	measles, mumps and rubella
MRI	magnetic resonance imaging
NF	neurofibromatosis
NICE	National Institute for Health and Clinical Excellence
NMSC	non-melanoma skin cancer
NSAID	non-steroidal anti-inflammatory drug
OCD	obsessive–compulsive disorder
PASI	psoriasis area and severity index
PCR	polymerase chain reaction
PCT	porphyria cutanea tarda
PDT	photodynamic therapy
PLE	polymorphic light eruption
PUVA	psoralen and ultraviolet A
PVL	Panton–Valentine leukocidin
QALY	quality adjusted life year
RAST	radioallergosorbent test
SCC	squamous cell carcinoma
SCORAD	SCORing Atopic Dermatitis
SJS	Stevens–Johnson syndrome
SLE	systemic lupus erythematosus
SPF	sun protection factor
SSMM	superficial spreading malignant melanoma
SSSS	staphylococcal scalded skin syndrome
STI	sexually transmitted infection
TB	tuberculosis
TEN	toxic epidermal necrolysis
UP	urticaria pigmentosa
UV	ultraviolet
UVR	ultraviolet radiation
VP	variegate porphyria
XP	xeroderma pigmentosa

1 Evidence based dermatology

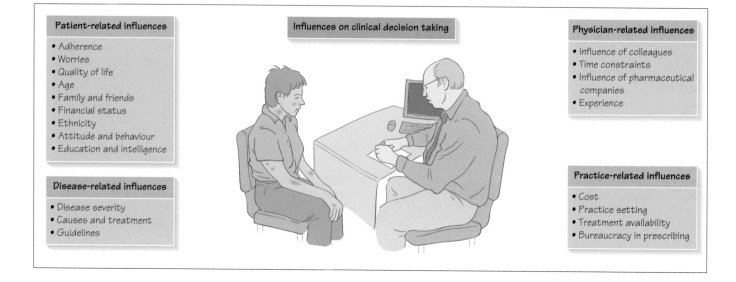

Influences on clinical decision taking

Patient-related influences
- Adherence
- Worries
- Quality of life
- Age
- Family and friends
- Financial status
- Ethnicity
- Attitude and behaviour
- Education and intelligence

Disease-related influences
- Disease severity
- Causes and treatment
- Guidelines

Physician-related influences
- Influence of colleagues
- Time constraints
- Influence of pharmaceutical companies
- Experience

Practice-related influences
- Cost
- Practice setting
- Treatment availability
- Bureaucracy in prescribing

Influences on clinical decision making

Drug prescription statistics across Europe show that there are vast differences in drug usage in dermatology from country to country. The diseases and the science of medicine are the same, but prescribing practice is hugely influenced by local custom and experience, habit and prejudices. There must be something wrong.

Clinical decision taking is very complex and a huge range of issues influence the clinician (Figure 1). But the foundation of high quality decision taking should be evidence based scientific information about the disease and its possible treatment.

Much of the management advice given in this book is not evidence based. Some may later be shown to be incorrect. Although the authors have tried to give evidence based information, this book gives their current opinions and some of their biases. So how could this be improved? How can clinical practice become based more on evidence and less on opinion?

Guidelines

It is helpful to have the well thought out views of others available in an easily digested form to guide you over therapy. Until recently, guidelines in dermatology and across the rest of medicine were usually written by a small group of self-appointed 'experts' who reached a consensus in discussion, based on their current practice. The likelihood of bias or missing the results of recent research was obvious. Over the last decade there has been a revolution in guideline writing. The processes are now designed to be structured and open. There is a formal literature review and guidelines are based on all the available evidence. When published, the strength of evidence backing up each recommendation is given. There is an open process of wide consultation before final acceptance and publication, and a date for review is set, usually after 3 or 4 years.

If you read any guidelines, make sure that their production was rigorous and evidence based, such as the British Association of Dermatologists' (BAD) guidelines (www.bad.org.uk) or the European Dermatology Forum guidelines (www.euroderm.org).

Systematic reviews

A systematic review is a very detailed structured literature review that aims to answer a specific research or therapy question. By having clear criteria for papers that will or will not be included and by searching very widely for all possible papers, it is possible to be confident in the results of such reviews. The study results may be combined by a process of meta-analysis. The Cochrane Group, named after a Cardiff chest physician and epidemiologist, coordinates and publishes these reviews: the Cochrane Skin Group reviews are at http://skin.cochrane.org.

UK Clinical Trials Network

If a drug really works dramatically then the numbers required to treat to prove effectiveness are very small. Only a handful of patients were needed to demonstrate that isotretinoin works in severe acne. But most advances in treatment are of smaller additional benefit and large double blind trials are essential.

The problem is that there are over 2000 different skin diseases: a dermatologist may only see some of these once every few years. It is impossible in a single centre to carry out prospective double blind trials on such uncommon conditions. It is also very costly. Many important clinical questions therefore remain unanswered.

So what can be done? The UK Dermatology Clinical Trials Network was set up by the Centre for Evidence Based Dermatology at Nottingham University, led by Professor Hywel Williams. The Network allows large numbers of dermatologists across the UK to contribute to high quality clinical studies of less common conditions to try to get some answers.

> **Key points**
> - Clinical decisions should ideally be based on evidence.
> - Systematic reviews identify current evidence and knowledge gaps.

Dermatology at a Glance, First Edition. Mahbub M.U. Chowdhury, Ruwani P. Katugampola, and Andrew Y. Finlay.

2 Dermatology: the best on the web

Free open access journals

Acta Dermato-Venereologica: www.medicaljournals.se/acta

BMC Dermatology: www.biomedcentral.com/bmcdermatol

Dermatology Online Journal: http://dermatology.cdlib.org

Many others at Directory of Open Access Journals: www.doaj.org

Detailed information about skin diseases

American Academy of Dermatology: www.aad.org/skin-conditions

New Zealand Dermatological Society (DermNet NZ): http://dermnetnz.org

Dermatology images

DermIS: Universities of Heidelberg and Erlangen: www.dermis.net

Global Skin Atlas: www.globalskinatlas.com

Interactive Medical Media (US company): www.dermnet.com

Paediatric Dermatology: DeBusk Dermatology Atlas: www.peds.ufl.edu/PEDS2/research/debusk/index.html

Clinical guidelines

British Association of Dermatologists. Evidence based guidelines >25 topics: www.bad.org.uk//site/622/default.aspx

European Guidelines: European Dermatology Forum >23 topics: www.euroderm.org

Quality of Life questionnaires, including DLQI

Department of Dermatology and Wound Healing, Cardiff University: www.dermatology.org.uk/quality/quality-life.html

Evidence based dermatology

Centre for Evidence Based Dermatology, Nottingham University: www.nottingham.ac.uk/scs/divisions/evidencebaseddermatology

Cochrane Skin Group: evidence based dermatology reviews: http://skin.cochrane.org

NHS Evidence: http://www2.evidence.nhs.uk

UK Dermatology Clinical Trials Network: www.ukdctn.org

Patient support groups

AcneNet American Academy of Dermatology Acne information: www.skincarephysicians.com/acnenet

British Association of Dermatologists list >60 UK groups: www.bad.org.uk//site/575/default.aspx

Changing Faces: www.changingfaces.org.uk

National Eczema Society: www.eczema.org/index.php

Psoriasis Association: www.psoriasis-association.org.uk

Vitiligo Society: www.vitiligosociety.org.uk

Patient information leaflets

British Association of Dermatologists. >120 leaflets: www.bad.org.uk/site/792/default.aspx

Patient information from BBC Health. >55 conditions: www.bbc.co.uk/health/physical_health/conditions/index.shtml?skin_disorders

Medical students

BAD Undergraduate Essay Prize, and BAD Undergraduate Dermatology Project/Elective Grants: www.bad.org.uk/site/619/default.aspx

Chiang, N. and Verbov, J. (2009) Dermatology: A handbook for medical students and junior doctors. British Association of Dermatologists (BAD) [70 page free book on-line aimed at UK medical students. Search full title of book on Google.]

Dermatology meetings: DermSchool: British Association of Dermatologists (BAD): www.bad.org.uk/site/616/default.aspx

Dermatology revision notes. Almost a doctor.com. http://almostadoctor.co.uk/content/systems/dermatology

Rees J. A Textbook of Skin Cancer and its Mimics. [Free book on-line aimed at medical students]. http://skincancer909.com

Dermatology news and reference

Medscape: US based news and reference: http://reference.medscape.com/dermatology

Dermatology quiz

Thirty cases with photos and answers from Melbourne, Australia: www.dermvic.org

Short video and sound lectures

Dermtube.com

Interactive Medical Media (US company): www.dermnet.com/videos.cfm

e-learning sample sessions

Department of Health and BAD project: two open access sessions: www.e-lfh.org.uk/projects/dermatology/sample_sessions.html

Free iPhone apps

Dermoscopy: Rao Dermatology: learn the basics of dermoscopy to aid pigmented lesion diagnosis.

Dermoscopy Tutorial. Genomel.

iABCD rule: Minidexs: diagnostic aid for malignant melanoma.

Psoriasis: Digital Lynx Ltd. PASI calculator to measure psoriasis.

PsoriasisTx. Advancing psoriasis and psoriatic arthritis management: Curatio CME Institute.

PubMed On Tap Lite.

SCORAD Index Linkwave. Measure Eczema (calculator in English).

Skin and Allergy news: the latest dermatology news.

Dermatology postgraduate distance learning course

Diploma and MSc in Practical Dermatology, Cardiff University: www.dermatology.org.uk

Dermatology at a Glance, First Edition. Mahbub M.U. Chowdhury, Ruwani P. Katugampola, and Andrew Y. Finlay.
© 2013 John Wiley & Sons, Ltd. Published 2013 by John Wiley & Sons, Ltd. **11**

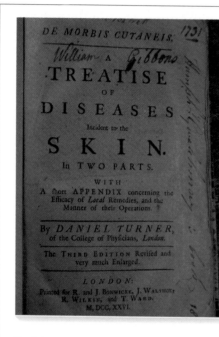

Fig. 3.1
Frontispiece of the first dermatology textbook in English, 1726 edition, by Daniel Turner

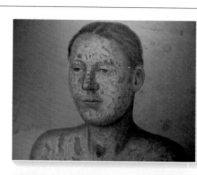

Fig. 3.2
Pemphigus foliaceus, from *Atlas of Skin Diseases,* Sydenham Society, late 19th Century

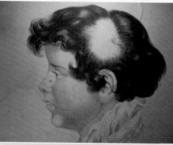

Fig. 3.3
Alopecia areata, from *Atlas of Skin Diseases,* Sydenham Society, late 19th Century

Fig. 3.4
Cleopatra's needle under restoration, transported to London in 1877 by Sir Erasmus Wilson

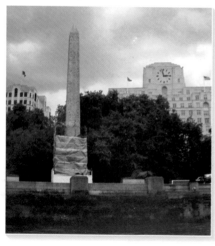

Fig. 3.5
Dr John Pringle (1855-1923), who described adenoma sebaceum, 'Pringle's disease'

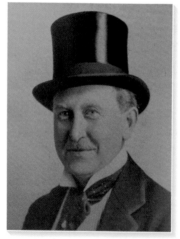

Fig. 3.6
Lupus vulgaris and cutaneous horn, from John Pringle's 1903 translation of Jacobi's *Portfolio of Dermochromes*

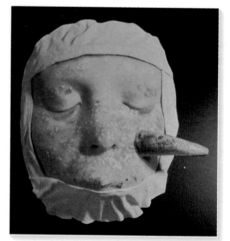

Table 3.1 **Key figures of 20th Century dermatology**

Sir Archibald Grey (1880-1967): founded the British Association of Dermatologists in 1921

Dr Geoffrey Dowling (1891-1976): an exceptional clinician and clear thinker who influenced a generation of British dermatologists

Dr Frederic Mohs (1910-2002): first used histologically controlled removal of skin cancer in 1936 in Wisconsin. The technique was named after him and is described in Chapter 9

Dr Albert Kligman (1916-2010): US dermatologist whose career spanned the introduction of topical steroids to the recognition of topical retinoids being effective in photodamage, a word he invented. Controversial because of his use of prisoners in clinical testing in the 1950's and 1960's

Dr Arthur Rook (1918-1991): a consultant first in Cardiff then in Cambridge, founded the Textbook of Dermatology, now the massive four volume standard textbook used by dermatologists worldwide

Dermatology at a Glance, First Edition. Mahbub M.U. Chowdhury, Ruwani P. Katugampola, and Andrew Y. Finlay.

Historical highlights

1572: The first printed book on dermatology, *De Morbis Cutaneis,* was published by Geronimo Mercuriali. He later presided over a disastrous medical response to the plague in Venice in 1576.

Eighteenth century: Dermatology emerges as a specialty. Skin diseases were usually dealt with by general physicians. Daniel Turner (1667–1740) trained as a surgeon, but in 1712 published the first skin disease book in English, *A Treatise of Diseases Incident to the Skin*, with detailed treatment recipes (Figure 3.1).

Eighteenth and nineteenth centuries: Classification war. Across science there was a huge drive to classify, in dermatology led by Joseph Plenck (1735–1807) from Vienna. Rival French and English classifications of skin disease were published; Robert Willan's (1757–1812) system (based on Plenck's) eventually won. Many of the disease names are still in use, including their mistakes (e.g. mycosis fungoides meaning 'fungus fungus', now known to be a T-cell lymphoma). Willan first described erythema nodosum.

Thomas Bateman (1778–1821) described molluscum contagiosum, alopecia areata and senile purpura. Clinical illustrations from the *Sydenham Society Atlas* (Figures 3.2 and 3.3) are still accurate.

Nineteenth century: German, Austrian and French dominance. Many skin diseases are named after the French or German dermatologists who first described them. Von Hebra (1816–1880) founded the influential Vienna Dermatology School and discovered the cause of scabies. In London, Erasmus Wilson (1809–1884), founded the *Journal of Cutaneous Medicine* and brought Cleopatra's Needle from Egypt to London (Figure 3.4). John Pringle described adenoma sebaceum (Figures 3.5, 3.6).

The golden age of skin hospitals. There were large numbers of dermatology beds. Often ineffective topical treatment was used for psoriasis, fungal disease, syphilis and tuberculosis.

Twentieth century (Table 3.1)
1903: Neils Finsen was awarded the Nobel Prize for UVB treatment of lupus vulgaris (skin tuberculosis).
1920: X-rays used for fungal skin infections and skin cancer.
1930–1950: Antibiotics conquer fatal cellulitis and tuberculosis. Goeckerman (tar + UVB) and Ingram regimes (dithranol + UVB) widely used for psoriasis.
1940: 'Dermatology and Venereology' grew as a single specialty as the skin and mucosal problems of syphilis and gonorrhoea were so common. But in the Second World War specialists treated sexually transmitted disease in the troops and the speciality of genito-urinary medicine developed from this. In Europe, only the UK, Eire and Malta have dermatology and venereology as separate specialities.
1950: Topical steroids: the biggest ever advance for eczema.
1960: Griseofulvin for fungal infection.
1970: PUVA for psoriasis, and topical azoles for fungal infection.
1980: Isotretinoin cures severe acne and ichthyoses controlled with etretinate or acitretin. Aciclovir introduced for herpes simplex.
AIDS: explosion of skin disease until retrovirals introduced.
1990: Terbinafine and itraconazole finally cure fungal infections.
Ciclosporin for psoriasis, after psoriasis improvement noticed after transplantation. New insight into its immunopathogenesis.

Twenty-first century

- Biologics for psoriasis revolutionise treatment of severe psoriasis, drastically reducing need for dermatology beds.
- Development of daycare treatment centres across the UK.
- Dermatology cancer therapy becomes major part of speciality.
- New subspecialities develop: cancer surgery, cutaneous allergy, photodermatology, paediatric dermatology, genital dermatology.
- Cosmetic dermatology grows rapidly in response to consumer/patient demand and new procedures (e.g. laser treatment).

The spreading of knowledge

British Journal of Dermatology (BJD): Founded in 1888 by Malcolm Morris and Henry Brooke, the *BJD* is one of the top dermatology journals worldwide. In 1921 Sir Archibald Grey and the *BJD* team founded the British Association of Dermatologists.

Journal of Investigative Dermatology: The highest impact scientific dermatology journal, official journal of the main European, American and Japanese scientific dermatology societies.

World Congress of Dermatology: Held every 5 years since the first in Paris in 1889, in London in 1896 and 1952. Now 4-yearly: Seoul 2011, Vancouver 2015.

Skin disease: cultural aspects

Films: www.SKinema.com describes:
- Actors with skin conditions (e.g. Tom Cruise and acne)
- Villains with skin conditions (e.g. Al Pacino in *Scarface*)
- Realistic roles of ordinary people with skin disease.

Television: The TV series *The Singing Detective*, a musical drama by Dennis Potter, was a focused portrayal of the anguish of severe psoriasis; Potter had psoriatic arthropathy. There were 240 references to dermatology in the 180 episodes of the comedy series *Seinfeld*, many depicting skin disease in a negative way.

Literature: Psoriasis in literature is well reviewed by Frans Meulenberg (*BMJ* 1997; 315:1709–11). John Updike had psoriasis, as did the main characters of *From the Journal of a Leper* and the novel *The Centaur*. Vladimir Nabokov (author of *Lolita*) had psoriasis but mostly ignored it in his writings. In *The Unconsoled* Kazuo Ishiguro describes a man with severe skin disease.

Art: Paul Klee (1879–1940), modern artist, had scleroderma, altering the way he used a paintbrush. There appears to be a basal cell carcinoma beneath Michelangelo's (1475–1564) eye in one of his self-portraits. In the *Mona Lisa* (1503) by Leonardo da Vinci, the yellow spot at the medial aspect of the left upper eyelid may be a xanthelasma: have a close look next time you are in Paris.

Pop music: Michael Jackson (1958–2009) stated in 1993 that he had vitiligo. His skin colour dramatically lightened.

Politics: The President of Ukraine, Viktor Yushchenko, was poisoned by dioxin in 2004. His face became disfigured by chloracne, with cysts and hyperpigmentation. Hidradenitis suppurativa had a major psychological effect on Karl Marx (1818–1883).

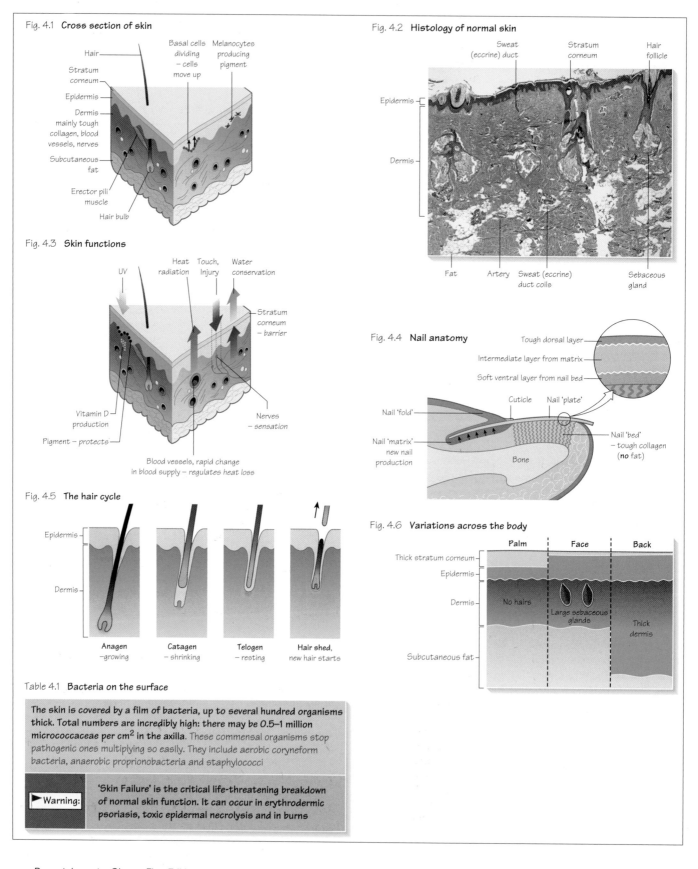

Fig. 4.1 **Cross section of skin**

Hair
Stratum corneum
Epidermis
Dermis mainly tough collagen, blood vessels, nerves
Subcutaneous fat
Erector pili muscle
Hair bulb
Basal cells dividing – cells move up
Melanocytes producing pigment

Fig. 4.2 **Histology of normal skin**

Sweat (eccrine) duct
Stratum corneum
Hair follicle
Epidermis
Dermis
Fat
Artery
Sweat (eccrine) duct coils
Sebaceous gland

Fig. 4.3 **Skin functions**

UV
Heat radiation
Touch, Injury
Water conservation
Stratum corneum – barrier
Vitamin D production
Pigment – protects
Nerves – sensation
Blood vessels, rapid change in blood supply – regulates heat loss

Fig. 4.4 **Nail anatomy**

Tough dorsal layer
Intermediate layer from matrix
Soft ventral layer from nail bed
Nail 'fold'
Cuticle
Nail 'plate'
Nail 'matrix' new nail production
Bone
Nail 'bed' – tough collagen (**no** fat)

Fig. 4.5 **The hair cycle**

Epidermis
Dermis
Anagen –growing
Catagen – shrinking
Telogen – resting
Hair shed, new hair starts

Fig. 4.6 **Variations across the body**

Palm
Face
Back
Thick stratum corneum
Epidermis
Dermis
Subcutaneous fat
No hairs
Large sebaceous glands
Thick dermis

Table 4.1 **Bacteria on the surface**

The skin is covered by a film of bacteria, up to several hundred organisms thick. Total numbers are incredibly high: there may be 0.5–1 million micrococcaceae per cm^2 in the axilla. These commensal organisms stop pathogenic ones multiplying so easily. They include aerobic coryneform bacteria, anaerobic proprionobacteria and staphylococci

▶ Warning: 'Skin Failure' is the critical life-threatening breakdown of normal skin function. It can occur in erythrodermic psoriasis, toxic epidermal necrolysis and in burns

Critical role of evolution

Without the stratum corneum, a highly effective waterproof layer, the body would rapidly dry out and die. But the skin, at the surface between inside and out, is maximally vulnerable to trauma.

Evolution's brilliant solution is to constantly replace the stratum corneum, with a feedback mechanism so that if there is any damage, replacement rate is rapidly stepped up. Various cell 'layers' are described in the epidermis, but in reality the epidermis is dynamic. There is a constant flow of new cells produced above the dermo-epidermal junction that flatten to form the stratum corneum when they reach the top, giving a new stratum corneum every month.

Ultraviolet protection

Ultraviolet (UV) radiation from the sun can cause dermal damage and promote skin cancer. Melanocytes, positioned above the dermo-epidermal junction, produce melanin in response to UV, resulting in temporary darkening, a tan. The high concentration of melanin in the deeply black skin of many African peoples provides very effective protection, whereas white skin in Northern climes allowed meagre sun exposure to be sufficient for vitamin D production.

Heat regulation

The blood flow through the dermis can be rapidly altered by valves regulating blood flow through capillaries in the upper dermis or by short-circuiting blood through dermal arterio-venous anastomoses.

If the core body temperature goes up, say during strenuous exercise, the amount of blood near the surface is massively increased, so heat radiates away from the body. The skin looks redder (flushed) because there is so much blood near the surface. If the core temperature remains too high, the sweat glands are turned on and the latent heat of evaporation results in some cooling.

If the core body temperature drops, blood supply to the skin surface is shut off. So the skin looks pale and feels cool. If this skin response is not sufficient to increase the core temperature, shivering starts and erector pili muscles contract ('goose pimples'), in a prehistoric but ineffective effort to increase the insulation.

Sensory

The range of different skin sensations includes touch, soreness, pain, itch, tickle, heat, cold and pressure. There is an obvious protective function, for example immediate withdrawal of a hand after feeling a dangerously hot area. These skin sensors provide critical interfaces between the body and the external world. Confirmation of limb positioning, intimate caressing and fine finger activities such as typing all depend on correctly functioning skin sensations.

Vitamin D production

Vitamin D is essential for calcium and phosphate regulation. Lack of vitamin D causes rickets, poorly formed bone, typically with curved tibia, or osteomalacia. Vitamin D is in the diet, mainly in milk and eggs, or is generated in the skin by ultraviolet B (UVB) from the sun acting on 7-dehydrocholesterol. This only happens outdoors, as UVB does not go through window glass. People with dark skin who live in the north and cover up their skin risk developing rickets.

Immunological functions

Langerhans cells in the epidermis are constantly on the alert for any unusual chemical touching the skin. New foreign chemicals are learnt by Langerhans cells, and information passed via the lymph nodes to circulating T cells. If the chemical is encountered again, a brisk inflammatory response is triggered, 'delayed hypersensitivity', attacking the unwanted antigen (see Chapter 30).

Sebaceous glands

The sebaceous glands are active from about 15 weeks *in utero*, but quickly become smaller at birth. They do not function again until puberty. Every hair follicle has a sebaceous gland attached to it. The glandular cells fall apart in the middle of the gland to produce the sebum (i.e. holocrine secretion). The sebum then lubricates the hair shaft and the surrounding skin. Sebum may have a protective function against bacteria and fungi.

Nails

- Fingernails are evolutionary remnants of our ancestors' claws.
- Nails are still important for fine manipulations such as untying knots or starting to peel an adhesive label.
- Most societies decorate nails and diseased nails can be a handicap in those jobs where normal looking hands are important.
- Nail is produced by the nail matrix (Figure 4.4). This consists of rapidly dividing specialised epidermal cells situated densely at the proximal end of each nail, protected by the overlying nail fold and cuticle.
- The epidermis under the nail contributes only minimally to new nail plate.
- Fingernails grow about 4 cm/year.

Regional variation and clinical relevance
(Figure 4.6)

- Facial skin contains very large sebaceous glands: acne, a disease of sebaceous glands, is most prominent on the face.
- Palmar and plantar skin has very thick stratum corneum with different keratin components. Genetic conditions such as tylosis (palmoplantar hyperkeratosis) can be confined to these sites.
- Where two skin surfaces come together in the body folds (flexures), the stratum corneum becomes moist and so a less efficient barrier. Superficial infections (e.g. intertrigo) occur and creams are absorbed more easily.
- The skin on the back is subject to extensive stress and has a thick dermis. Injury or surgery causes more obvious scarring.

Skin and hair colour

There is wide racial variation in the amount and type of pigment that is produced by melanocytes and then transferred to keratinocytes in the epidermis. The main dark pigments are eumelanins and the red–yellow pigments are phaeomelanins (seen in blond or pale skinned individuals). Red hair also contains intensely coloured trichochromes. Red and blonde haired people have a much higher lifetime risk of developing skin cancer.

Key points

- Skin has several critical functions essential to life.
- Severe disease results in skin failure, high morbidity or even death.

Fig. 5.1 The ripple effect

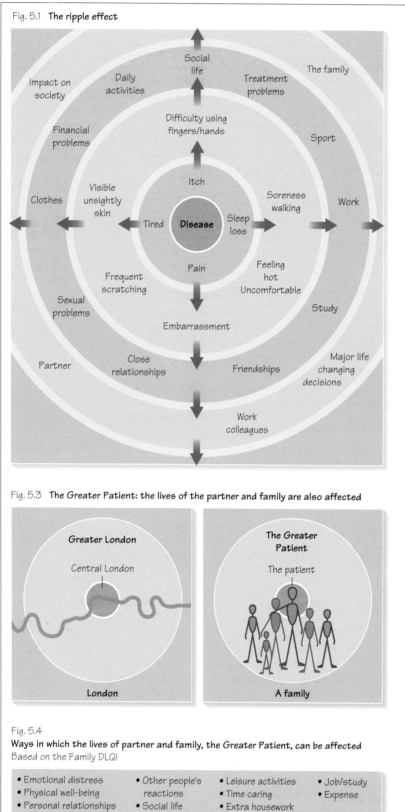

Impact on society · Daily activities · Social life · Treatment problems · The family

Financial problems · Difficulty using fingers/hands · Sport

Clothes · Visible unsightly skin · Itch · Soreness walking · Work

Tired · **Disease** · Sleep loss

Pain · Feeling hot Uncomfortable · Study

Sexual problems · Frequent scratching · Embarrassment

Partner · Close relationships · Friendships · Major life changing decisions

Work colleagues

Fig. 5.3 The Greater Patient: the lives of the partner and family are also affected

Greater London
Central London
London

The Greater Patient
The patient
A family

Fig. 5.4
Ways in which the lives of partner and family, the Greater Patient, can be affected
Based on the Family DLQI

- Emotional distress
- Physical well-being
- Personal relationships
- Other people's reactions
- Social life
- Leisure activities
- Time caring
- Extra housework
- Job/study
- Expense

Fig. 5.2
A question from the Children's Dermatology Life Quality Index
How much have you avoided swimming or other sports because of your skin trouble?

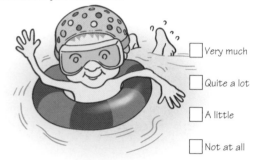

☐ Very much
☐ Quite a lot
☐ A little
☐ Not at all

Table 5.1
Measurement of quality of life impact of skin disease

Helpful in:
- Routine clinical practice
- Auditing effectiveness of a clinical service
- Assessing the value of a new drug
- Clinical research
- Arguing for more resources for dermatology services or research

Table 5.2
Dermatology Life Quality Index (DLQI) question topics

1. Symptoms: itchy, sore, pain, stinging
2. Embarrassment or self-conscious
3. Shopping, home, garden
4. Clothes
5. Social, leisure activities
6. Sport
7. Work, study
8. Partner, close friends or relatives
9. Sexual difficulties
10. Treatment problems

Every question relates to the last week and is scored 0–3, giving a maximum score of 30

To access the DLQI go to www.dermatology.org.uk
– full text, >80 translations (©AY Finlay, GK Khan, April 1992)

Table 5.3 How to understand DLQI scores

These are the validated score bands	0 – 1	no effect
	2 – 5	small effect
Overall impact on patient's life	6 – 10	moderate effect
	11 – 20	very large effect
	21 – 30	extremely large effect

Table 5.4 Learning Haiku

If their QoL score is ten or more, you can be sure life quality is poor

Dermatology at a Glance, First Edition. Mahbub M.U. Chowdhury, Ruwani P. Katugampola, and Andrew Y. Finlay.

How skin disease affects peoples' lives

Many patients with skin disease experience a major impact on their quality of life, although some continue their lives as normal (Figure 5.1). Chronic inflammatory skin diseases such as severe psoriasis, eczema, acne and hidradenitis suppurativa cause the greatest life quality impairment and disfiguring diseases such as vitiligo and alopecia areata also cause major problems. Virtually all aspects of patients' lives can be affected, including home care, shopping, choice of clothes, social activities, sport, study, work, personal and sexual relationships. Patients experience itchiness and embarrassment, and the treatment itself, especially if topical, can add to the burden.

Understanding patient's quality of life impact helps clinical practice

One of the main reasons that people seek help for their skin disease is that it is disrupting their lives. When taking clinical decisions in dermatology, clinicians are influenced by how severely they think the patient's life is affected. If you understand this impact accurately, your clinical decisions will be more appropriate. Simply ask 'How is your skin disease affecting your life at the moment?' Formal measurement with a quality of life questionnaire may be helpful (e.g. when considering prescribing a systemic therapy).

How to measure the impact of skin disease on life quality

There are dermatology-specific questionnaires such as the Dermatology Life Quality Index (DLQI) or Skindex, disease-specific questionnaires, such as the Psoriasis or Acne Disability Indices, and generic measures that can be used across all diseases (Table 5.1).

Comparison with non-skin diseases

It is important to be able to compare the impact on quality of life of a skin disease with a non-skin disease (e.g. diabetes or ulcerative colitis), so that the burden of skin disease is understood when decisions are being taken about health care resource allocation. Generic quality of life questionnaires such as the SF-36, EuroQol or WHO-BREV are used. Questions cover all the ways that diseases, across the whole of medicine, can affect people's lives. Severe psoriasis causes as much life quality impairment as diabetes or heart failure, using the SF-36.

Dermatology Life Quality Index

The DLQI (Tables 5.2 and 5.3) is used in many clinical research studies as a patient reported outcome measure to find out how effective treatments are, from the patient's point of view. This information complements the traditional measures of extent of disease or number of lesions, as the degree of impact experienced by a patient may not be predictable by examining the skin, but is strongly influenced by the patient's personality and attitudes, current circumstances and their experiences of the reaction of others to their skin problem.

Rule of Tens: using quality of life scores to help define disease severity

The Rule of Tens states that if a patient with psoriasis has:
- Body surface area affected >10% *or*
- PASI (psoriasis area and severity index score) >10 *or*
- DLQI (dermatology life quality index score) >10
then consider that the patient has severe psoriasis.

This indicates the need to consider aggressive therapy, possibly systemic. The Rule of Tens is used to guide the clinical decision whether biological therapies should be used in psoriasis.

Major life changing decisions

Skin disease not only affects patients now, but may have a profound influence on major life changing decisions, such as what career to follow, whether to have children or whether to move to another city or country. Having a skin disease may therefore have long-term repercussions on whole life development.

Children

Children's lives can also be severely disturbed by skin disease. School work, play, holiday activities and choice of clothes can all be affected. The simple 10-question Children's Dermatology Life Quality Index, available as a text or cartoon version, measures these effects (Figure 5.2).

The Greater Patient

If a patient has a skin disease, the lives of the patient's partner and family members may also be affected (Figure 5.3). The patient (at the centre) impacts on the Greater Patient (the partner and/or affected family members). Parents of a child with severe atopic dermatitis have sleep disturbed and family activities have to be curtailed; the partner of a man with severe psoriasis finds that her social and sexual life is affected. This secondary effect on the Greater Patient can be measured using the Family Dermatology Life Quality Index (Figure 5.4).

Utility measures

This is a way of 'converting' life impairment experienced by a patient into hypothetical cash, time or lifespan equivalents.

Example: 88% of people with acne attending a hospital clinic would rather have a cure for their acne than be given £500.

Quality adjusted life years (QALY) are used as a method of calculating the benefit of a treatment, so that the benefit can be compared with the benefit from other interventions and also with its cost.

Key points

- Try to understand both the patient's and the relative's experience and think of ways to improve their situation.
- Remember to use the routine question 'How much is your skin disease affecting your life at the moment?'
- Measurement of skin disease impact may help improve decisions.

▶ Warning

Don't rely on guesswork to understand how your patient's life is affected by the skin disease – ask!

6 Taking the history

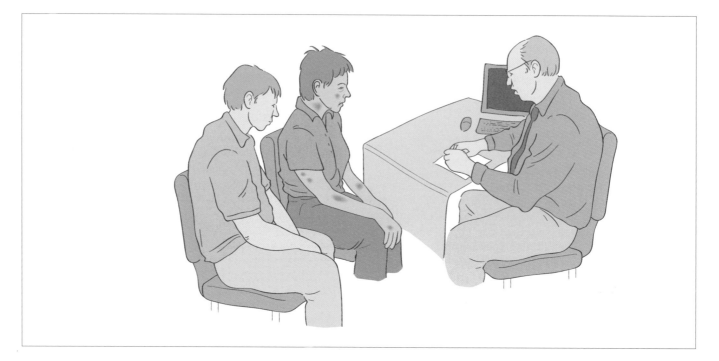

For the next few minutes, my only concern is the patient in this room. I won't let anything distract me, and I will focus and attend to this patient, making sure they feel cared for and respected. (Steven R. Feldman. *J Dermatol Treat* 2010; 21:217)

Why taking a history is important

Skin disease is very visible. Most doctors (despite protesting ignorance) can instantly diagnose several common skin diseases. There are several hundred rarer skin conditions that dermatologists rapidly recognise: this is one of the attractions and satisfactions of clinical dermatology. So why bother with a history?

• Taking an accurate history is at the heart of good medicine.
• If you don't take an accurate history you will miss vital information.
• You need to know about the previous history of the skin condition and its response to treatment to be able to judge what therapy should be suggested.
• You can't tell how much the patient's life is being affected by just examining the skin.
• You need to know what drugs the patient is taking because they may have caused or be making the skin condition worse.
• You need to know the family history in case there is a genetic aspect to the condition or in case the condition is infectious.
• You need to know about the impact of the patient's work on the skin condition and the influence of the skin condition on the patient's ability to work.
• You need to know about associated conditions such as atopic diseases or diabetes.
• You need to be able to assess the psychological impact of the disease. Is the patient depressed because of the skin problem?
• You need to know about the family to assess how much support is available for the treatment you may suggest.

Patients are eager to show you their skin problem straight away ('the rolled up trouser leg syndrome'). If so, look briefly but carefully and explain that you want to ask a few questions before you examine them fully.

Structured history taking

Introduction
• Use general open question (e.g. 'What is the problem?')

Current complaint
• When started?
• Course of disease (steady, intermittent)?
• Main symptoms?
• Which areas are affected?
• What makes it better or worse?

Past medical history
• Details of previous skin disease
• Ask about common skin diseases (e.g. eczema, psoriasis, acne)
• Ask about common systemic diseases with skin manifestations (e.g. diabetes, TB, immunosuppression and/or HIV)

Drugs and allergies
• Current topical and systemic drugs
• Other topical and systemic drugs used in the past for skin disease and their benefit
• History suggesting contact allergy (e.g. nickel, perfume)
• History of allergy to systemic drugs
• History of immediate allergy (e.g. latex)

Social history
• Current impact of skin disease on life and work?
• Impact of work on skin disease?
• Alcohol (alcoholism is a risk factor in worsening of psoriasis)?

Dermatology at a Glance, First Edition. Mahbub M.U. Chowdhury, Ruwani P. Katugampola, and Andrew Y. Finlay.

- Smoker (smoking is strongly associated with palmo-plantar pustulosis and hidradenitis suppurativa)?
- History of high sun exposure or sunbed use?

Family history
- Eczema, asthma, hay fever?
- Psoriasis?
- Genetic disease?
- Skin cancer?

Key points to a successful consultation
- Greet the patient by name and introduce yourself.
- Address the patient appropriately and respectfully. Do not assume that using the patient's first name will always make them feel at ease, it may be perceived as over familiar.
- Initially let the patient talk uninterrupted. Patients will talk only for a few minutes on average. This saves time later and the patient feels happy to have told you what is important to them.
- Listen to the patient.
- Repeat your understanding of the key information the patient has given you.
- Sit at the same height as the patient, at an angle, not divided by desk or computer.
- Have lots of eye contact with the patient.
- Check that the patient understands what you are saying to them.
- Seek permission from the patient for students to be present.

Special circumstances
Children
Although the main history comes from the parent, involve the child. Does the child really want treatment for that wart, or is it just the parent?

Elderly
The elderly usually need more time. Accept it. You may need to speak more slowly and clearly. The elderly may have their own ideas about what is best for them. Listen, they are often right.

Language and translations
If a person's English is so bad that they need a translator, look around the clinic staff and students for someone fluent. You may need to rebook the appointment when a translator can be there to ensure that you can communicate. When speaking through a translator still speak directly to the patient and also use sign 'language' to give your meaning directly to the patient.

Adolescents
- Try to empathise.
- Try to imagine what it is like for them, even though they appear to be rude or difficult.
- Speak to them, not to the parent.
- Indicate subtly that you are listening to them and taking their side when a disagreement breaks out with a parent.
- Be aggressive with treatment, show that you want them to get results.
- Be aware of potential major adherence problems.

History taking with experience
Experience will allow 'homing in' on critical relevant information. However, do not be over-confident: you still need to have a structure to ensure you do not miss relevant information.

Why recording the history is important
Clinical reasons
- To avoid repetitive history taking
- Quality control that you have covered all key aspects of history
- Clear record of current drugs and dosages
- Comparative purposes for future consultations

Medico-legal reasons
- Evidence that a careful history was taken
- Evidence that particular information was given

Multi-tasking in the clinic
Apart from the core business of history taking, patient examination and clinical decision taking, there are many demands on time in the clinic. You need to learn to address these but always place the patient at the centre of them.
- Seek permission for teaching, do not assume it.
- If you need to discuss matters with a colleague, explain to the patient why this may help them.
- You may need to answer a phone to silence it ringing, but explain to the caller that you will phone them back after the consultation.
- If you must take the call, ask the patient and explain why.
- The patient will approve of you seeking more information from books or online if you give a running commentary.
- Dictating letters about a patient in front of a patient can be very helpful to a consultation: the patient knows that the letter has definitely been written. You can check with the patient that what you are saying is accurate and the patient has the opportunity to flag up any mistakes.
- Manage clinic issues between patients, not during consultations.

How to take clinical decisions: the art of medicine
To take a clinical decision you need accurate information from a detailed history and examination. Decisions should be informed by scientific evidence. Local and national guidelines seek to provide evidence based guidelines based on the most reliable relevant science (see Chapter 1).

But there are many non-scientific influences on decision taking: some influences are good, others bad. Non-clinical influences are patient, clinician and practice related. Examples include where a patient lives, intelligence, age, personality, family members' influence, clinician time constraints, relationships with colleagues and prescribing bureaucracy. You need to be aware of these influences to ensure that your decision is best for that patient.

Processing patient information, scientific knowledge and the other influences constitutes the art of medicine: clinical medicine is complex, challenging and rewarding.

> **Key point**
>
> A structured history is essential for diagnosis and management.

> ▶ **Warning**
>
> Don't skimp on the history just because the disease is visible.

7 How to examine the skin

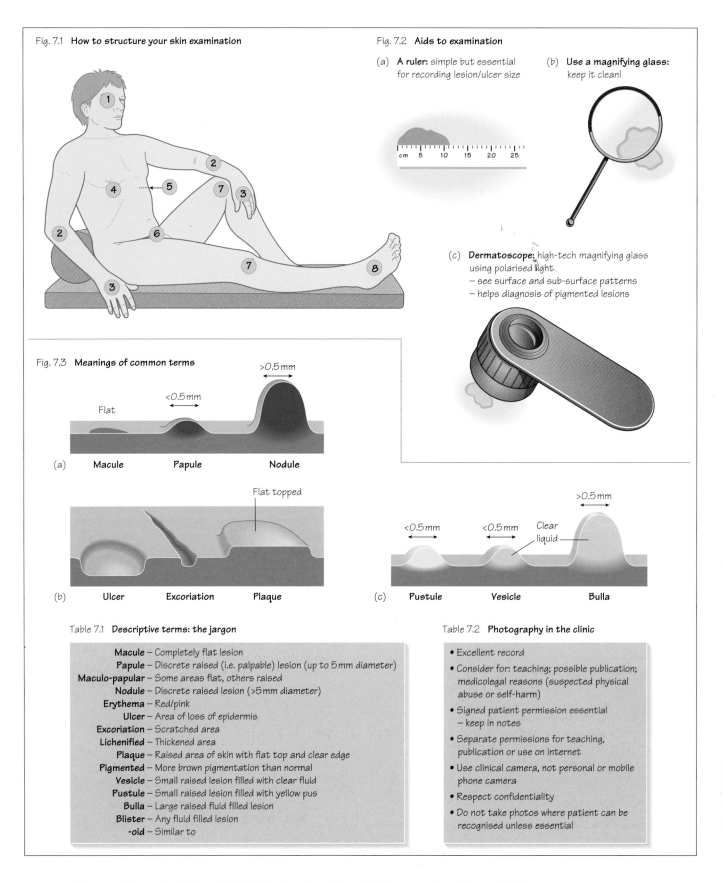

Fig. 7.1 How to structure your skin examination

Fig. 7.2 Aids to examination

(a) **A ruler:** simple but essential for recording lesion/ulcer size

(b) **Use a magnifying glass:** keep it clean!

(c) **Dermatoscope:** high-tech magnifying glass using polarised light
 – see surface and sub-surface patterns
 – helps diagnosis of pigmented lesions

Fig. 7.3 Meanings of common terms

(a) Macule   Papule   Nodule

Flat   <0.5mm   >0.5mm

(b) Ulcer   Excoriation   Plaque

Flat topped

(c) Pustule   Vesicle   Bulla

<0.5mm   <0.5mm   Clear liquid   >0.5mm

Table 7.1 Descriptive terms: the jargon

Macule	Completely flat lesion
Papule	Discrete raised (i.e. palpable) lesion (up to 5mm diameter)
Maculo-papular	Some areas flat, others raised
Nodule	Discrete raised lesion (>5mm diameter)
Erythema	Red/pink
Ulcer	Area of loss of epidermis
Excoriation	Scratched area
Lichenified	Thickened area
Plaque	Raised area of skin with flat top and clear edge
Pigmented	More brown pigmentation than normal
Vesicle	Small raised lesion filled with clear fluid
Pustule	Small raised lesion filled with yellow pus
Bulla	Large raised fluid filled lesion
Blister	Any fluid filled lesion
-oid	Similar to

Table 7.2 Photography in the clinic

- Excellent record
- Consider for: teaching; possible publication; medicolegal reasons (suspected physical abuse or self-harm)
- Signed patient permission essential – keep in notes
- Separate permissions for teaching, publication or use on internet
- Use clinical camera, not personal or mobile phone camera
- Respect confidentiality
- Do not take photos where patient can be recognised unless essential

Dermatology at a Glance, First Edition. Mahbub M.U. Chowdhury, Ruwani P. Katugampola, and Andrew Y. Finlay.
© 2013 John Wiley & Sons, Ltd. Published 2013 by John Wiley & Sons, Ltd.

Examination optimal conditions

First you need to get the patient in the best position to be examined:
- Privacy
- Chaperone
- Patient undressed
- On a couch
- Bright light

Essential (Figure 7.2)
- Willingness to examine the patient properly
- Thinking seeing (not just looking)
- Ruler handy
- Magnifying glass and dermatoscope available

Simple structure

You need a simple structure to make sure that you have seen all the skin. 'Start at the top and work your way down' (Figure 7.1).

Scalp
- Think about the scalp and the hair separately
- Feel the scalp as the hair may be too thick to see much
- Part the hair to see the scalp
- Pick up hair at the edge of the scalp to see the edge of the rash (e.g. psoriasis)
- Any baldness? If yes, any alopecia areata 'exclamation mark' hairs (see Chapter 25)?
- Any scarring (flat shiny bald areas free of follicle openings)?
- Any unusual hair thickness or twistiness?

Ears
External pinnae
- Signs of solar damage especially at the edge
- Scaliness suggesting seborrhoeic dermatitis
- Discrete tender area on prominent ridge suggesting chondrodermatitis

External auditory meatus
- Psoriasis
- Eczema

Face
- Examine areas of maximum sun damage: forehead, upper cheeks and nose. Any sign of skin cancer?
- Hair growth normal (also eyelashes, eyebrows)?
- Eyes: mucosal surfaces
- Lips, mouth: check tongue, gums and buccal mucosal surface inside cheeks (e.g. white net-like pattern of lichen planus)

Neck, axillae and arms
Flexures
- Axillae: erythrasma, hidradenitis suppurativa, fungal infection, flexural psoriasis, seborrhoeic dermatitis?
- Antecubital fossae: atopic eczema?

Extensors
- Elbows: psoriasis?

Hands
- Wrists: scabies?
- Finger webs: irritant contact dermatitis, scabies?
- Nails: fungal infection, psoriasis?

Trunk: back, chest, abdomen and buttocks
- Upper trunk: acne?
- Flexures: intertrigo?
- Nipples: atopic eczema, contact dermatitis, Paget's disease?
- Umbilicus: psoriasis?

Genitalia, perineum, groins and peri-anal skin
- Contact dermatitis
- Fungal infection
- Intertrigo
- Genital warts or discharge

Legs
- Flexures: atopic eczema?
- Knees: psoriasis?
- Lower legs: varicose veins?
- Ankles: venous eczema?

Feet
- Soles: pustular psoriasis?
- Toe webs: fungal infection?
- Toenails: fungal infection, onychogryphosis?

General points: all areas
- Hair growth pattern normal?
- Hair pigmentation normal?
- Skin pigmentation normal?
- Condition symmetrical?
- Sun damage pattern (differences covered–uncovered areas)?

Individual lesions (Figure 7.3)
- Where?
- Size: diameter?
- Colour? Variable pigment?
- Raised or flat?
- Edge: smooth or irregular?

Recording examination findings
- Essential for later comparison and for medico-legal reasons
- Write down immediately main positive and negative findings
- Record lesion measurements immediately

Special situations
- Patient shy or refuses examination
- Chaperone essential
- Try to understand patient's concern: religious, cultural, personality?
- Explain why examination is essential to provide best advice
- Sometimes patients allow examination of only one or more limited areas
- If permission refused, record this but still try to provide advice, with caveats

> **Key points**
>
> - Remember to 'start at the top, and work your way down'.
> - Keep clear records of history and examination.

> ► **Warning**
>
> - It's tempting to only look at the skin areas mentioned by the patient.
> - If you don't examine the skin fully, you may make the wrong diagnosis or prescribe the wrong treatment.

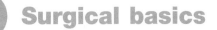

Table 8.1 Pre-surgical counselling

- Obtain formal verbal or written informed consent
- Explain risks e.g. infection, bleeding, nerve damage, pigment change
- Warn regarding type of scar and risk of keloid e.g. on chest, shoulder
- Warn regarding limitation of use of limbs and/or time off work

Table 8.2

Surgery procedures used in dermatology

- Shave biopsy
- Punch biopsy
- Curettage
- Incisional biopsy
- Excision

Fig. 8.1 Anatomy of the face to show location of branches of the facial nerve in relation to the fascia and parotid gland, and the overlying facial and superficial temporal arteries

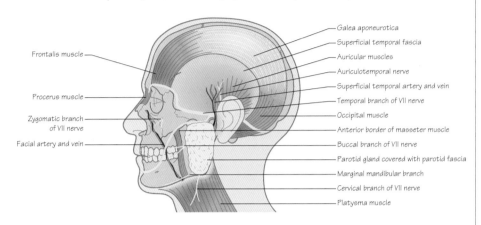

Frontalis muscle
Procerus muscle
Zygomatic branch of VII nerve
Facial artery and vein

Galea aponeurotica
Superficial temporal fascia
Auricular muscles
Auriculotemporal nerve
Superficial temporal artery and vein
Temporal branch of VII nerve
Occipital muscle
Anterior border of masseter muscle
Buccal branch of VII nerve
Parotid gland covered with parotid fascia
Marginal mandibular branch
Cervical branch of VII nerve
Platysma muscle

(Figs 8.1, 8.4 and 8.6 from Finlay AY, Chowdhury MMU (eds) (2007). Specialist Training in Dermatology, reproduced with permission of Elsevier)

Fig. 8.2 Benign mole removed with half blade and haemostatic applied with cotton bud leaving a circular defect

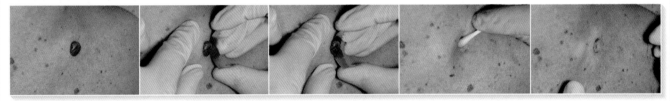

Fig. 8.3
(a) **4 mm punch biopsy**
(b) **Punch biopsy on cheek**

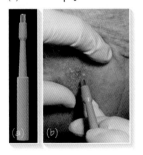

Fig. 8.4
Punch biopsy: stretch the skin (a), at right angles to the intended direction of the scar (b), remove the biopsy by cutting (c), do not crush the specimen. The defect (d) is then sutured (e)

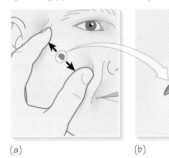

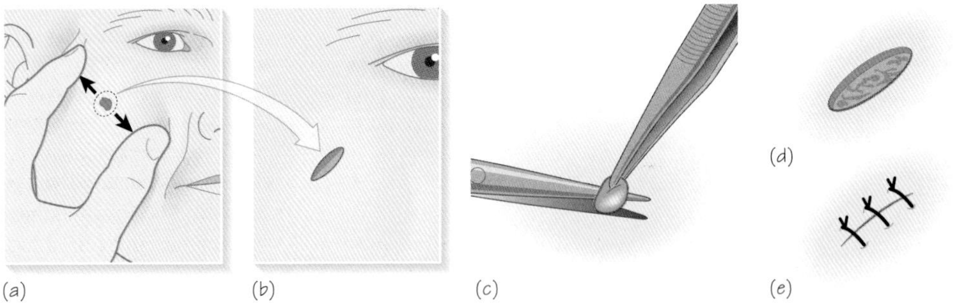

(a) (b) (c) (d) (e)

Fig. 8.5
(a) **Curette**
(b) **Curette with sharp margin used on cheek**

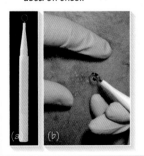

Fig. 8.6
Types of skin biopsies

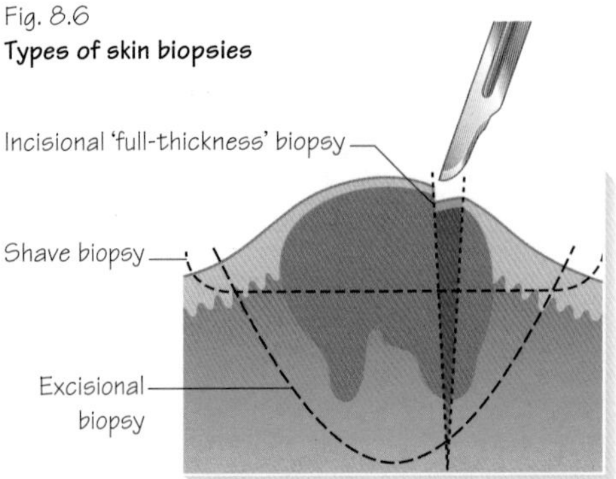

Incisional 'full-thickness' biopsy
Shave biopsy
Excisional biopsy

Fig. 8.7
Skin tumour marked with 5 mm margin and ready for full ellipse excision

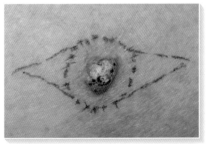

The ability to perform some basic surgery is an essential part of a dermatologist's skills and many GPs now also undertake simple procedures. Up to 60% of referrals to Dermatology may need some surgical intervention.

Preparation prior to surgery

Full counselling is essential prior to any surgical procedure to explain why the procedure is necessary, what will be done and possible complications (Table 8.1). This avoids any conflict and potential complaints afterwards.

Pre-operative history should include past medical history and drug history including anti-coagulants and anti-platelets (e.g. warfarin, aspirin) which may need to be stopped prior to surgery.

Basic understanding of anatomy is essential to perform surgery safely, particularly on the face and neck (e.g. branches of the facial nerve and superficial temporal arteries need to be avoided; Figure 8.1).

Local anaesthesia

1% or 2% lidocaine is used with adrenaline (1 : 80,000 or 1 : 200,000) or without adrenaline. A person weighing 70 kg can have a maximum of 50 mL 1% lidocaine with 1 : 200,000 adrenaline. Adrenaline causes vasoconstriction to reduce bleeding and also increases the duration of the anaesthesia.

Use lidocaine with caution in patients taking non-selective beta-blockers as this can lead to hypertension and reflex bradycardia.

Nerve blocks use less volume and can give effective anaesthesia (e.g. supra/infraorbital). Digital ring blocks for finger anaesthesia usually use plain lidocaine without adrenaline to reduce the risk of ischaemia.

The pain of local anaesthetic injections can be reduced (e.g. in children) with the use of tetracaine gel (Ametop®) used 30 minutes pre-operatively. Other tricks include using 0.5% plain lidocaine without preservative with a small gauge (30 g) needle followed by 1% lidocaine with 1 : 200,000 adrenaline.

Always check the anaesthetic has been effective before starting the procedure!

Side effects of local anaesthetic include accidental injection and toxicity, pain and temporary weakness of muscles (e.g. difficulty raising the eyebrows or closing the eyes after injecting the temple area).

Haemostasis

Solutions such as 20% aluminium chloride and 20% isopropyl alcohol or silver nitrate are used to stop bleeding in simple procedures (e.g. shave biopsy). Other options include electrocautery (current passing through high resistance metal), which produces heat with the cautery tip applied lightly to the wound surface. Avoid alcohol-based antiseptics when using this method because of the risk of fire.

Diathermy also generates heat by resistance to current which passes through the tissues. The use of the diathermy may include deliberate sparking with superficial damage to the skin and light scarring. If direct contact is made with the skin with the diathermy tip then the heat is produced at a deeper level and is more likely to cause scarring.

Deeper wounds can have firm pressure around the edge of the wound to stop bleeding and then be sealed with diathermy, or an absorbable suture is tied around the vessel. Electrocoagulation (bipolar AC current) can be used for deeper wounds with the current applied to the tissue by the forceps through to the vessel causing necrosis. Care must be taken with electrosurgery instruments because of possible pacemaker interference. This may need to be discussed in advance with the cardiologist.

Surgical procedures (Table 8.2)

Shave biopsy Local anaesthetic is injected subcutaneously under the lesion without elevation. The skin is stretched firmly. A razor blade or surgical blade is then moved to and fro under the lesion to remove it, leaving a flat surface (Figure 8.2).

Punch biopsy The skin is infiltrated with local anaesthetic around the area of biopsy. Stretch the skin at right angles to the preferred alignment of the scar (Figures 8.3 and 8.4). A 3–6 mm punch is rotated into the skin releasing the area of skin still attached to the base. This skin is lifted gently and cut beneath with sharp scissors. Suturing is with 6-0 polyamide (Ethilon®) on the face or 4-0 on the limbs. Sutures can be removed after 5–7 days for the face and 7–10 days for the trunk and limbs.

Curettage Disposable ring curettes that have a sharp and blunt side are used (Figure 8.5). The curette's sharp side is used to separate (scrape) the tumour from the underlying skin with a gentle regular sideways action under local anaesthetic.

Incisional biopsy This is used to diagnose inflammatory skin conditions, infiltrative disorders and skin cancers (e.g. panniculitis, vasculitis or squamous cell carcinoma). This technique allows histological examination of the dermis and dermal–fat interface. The skin is removed as a narrow but deep wedge and sutured as above (Figure 8.6).

Full excision This technique is used for full removal of skin tumours such as basal cell carcinoma, squamous cell carcinoma and melanoma. Awareness of skin tension lines allows prediction of the best surgical scar. The skin must be marked with a sterile pen prior to local anaesthetic use. Antiseptics such as chlorhexidine 0.05% aqueous or iodine solutions can be used.

Ellipse excision ideally has a length : breadth ratio of 3 : 1 (Figure 8.7). Sutures should enter and exit the wound perpendicular to the surface and surface sutures should have minimum tension. Subcutaneous sutures include vicryl (Ethicon®) and polydioxanone (PDS®). These retain 50% of their strength at 3–6 weeks postoperatively. Surface sutures include Ethilon® or Prolene® from 3-0 to 6-0 (finer suture).

A dressing such as iodine (Inadine®) overlying antibiotic ointment (Polyfax®) can be used. This is followed with application of white soft paraffin (Vaseline®) daily for 7–10 days once the dressing is removed to prevent the wound from drying and crusting which tends to leave a worse scar.

Key points

- Simple surgical procedures are now commonly undertaken for diagnosis and management.
- No surgery should be considered 'minor'.
- Give full explanation prior to the procedure.
- Warn all patients regarding possible complications such as bleeding, infection and scarring.

▶ Warning

Do not start the procedure unless the patient is 100% sure he or she wishes to proceed.

Table 9.1
Some procedures used in dermatology

- Cryotherapy
- Laser
- Botulinum toxin injections
- Iontophoresis (see Chapter 11)
- Trichloroacetic acid treatment
- Mohs' micrographic surgery
- Full thickness skin graft/flap repair
- Nail surgery

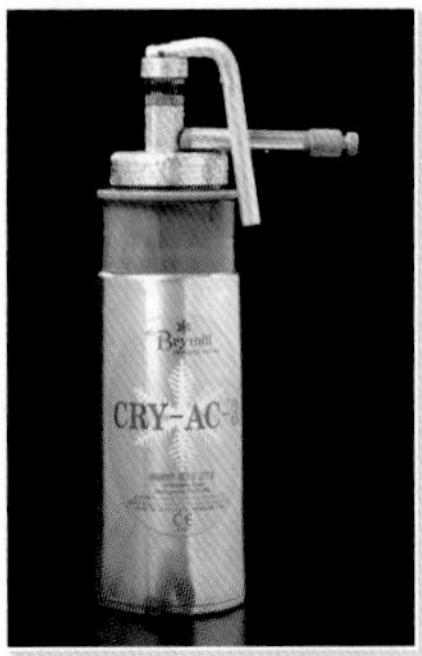

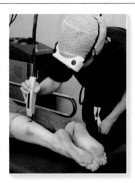

Fig. 9.1
Cryogun

Fig. 9.2
Pulse dye laser to treat vascular lesion on leg

Fig. 9.3a/b
Axillary hyperhidrosis treated with multiple botulinum toxin injections

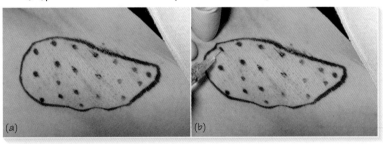

(a)   (b)

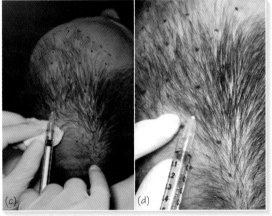

(c)   (d)

Fig. 9.3c/d
Botulinum toxin for scalp hyperhidrosis

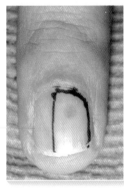

Fig. 9.4a
Glomus tumour under nail plate marked prior to surgery

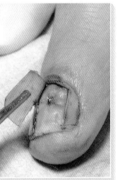

Fig. 9.4b
Nail reflected under ring block and biopsy taken of tumour

Fig. 9.5   Mohs' surgery.
The tumour is debulked with curettage. A thin plate encompassing the entire margin and wound bed is excised. The tissue is then divided into quadrants and the cut edges marked with dye. The surgical margin is sectioned horizontally to include the epidermis and deep margins and examined under the microscope. Any tumour seen has breached the surgical margin and can be located to the exact location in the wound (quadrant b in this case). Further tissue can be removed until the surgical margins are tumour free.

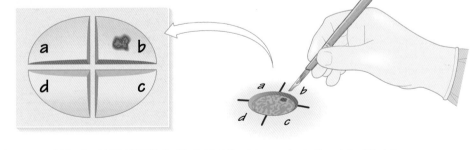

(Source: Finlay AY, Chowdhury MMU (eds) (2007). Specialist Training in Dermatology, reproduced with permission of Elsevier)

This chapter describes other key procedures that are used in dermatology as listed in Table 9.1.

Cryotherapy

Liquid nitrogen cryosurgery is the most common form of cryotherapy used, with temperatures reaching down to –30°C. This achieves destruction of the tissue.

The spray technique with a cryogun is easiest to use (Figure 9.1). The aim is to achieve an ice field quickly with the spray tip held up to 1 cm away from the skin surface. Freeze times vary, with 5–10 seconds used for viral warts, solar keratoses and seborrhoeic warts. Bowen's disease, superficial basal cell carcinomas (BCC) and small squamous cell carcinomas (SCC) can be treated with 30–60 seconds and a second refreeze after thawing.

Certain tumours are not suitable for treatment with cryotherapy (e.g. morphoeic BCC, large tumours >2 cm in diameter and ill-defined tumours).

Cryosurgery is painful and so young children less than 12 years of age may not tolerate it. Local anaesthetic can be used prior and two cycles of freezing may be needed in larger areas.

Side effects include pain, large blisters and swelling. If plantar warts are treated they may limit walking for a few days. Hyper and hypopigmentation can occur in patients with darker skin and hence may need to be avoided in this group.

Laser (light amplification by stimulated emission of radiation)

This has been used for many years in dermatology to treat vascular and pigmented lesions, scars, tattoos and increased hair growth. Laser treatments are frequently requested by patients so a basic understanding is useful.

Lasers currently used include CO_2, pulse dye (Figure 9.2) and erbium:YAG. The components of the laser include laser medium, optical cavity and pumping system. Atoms in the laser medium are excited by an external source of energy into an unstable state and electrons then returning to their resting state emit energy. This energy is emitted as light which travels as photons. These photons are reflected by mirrors allowing a portion of the light to travel out of the optical cavity as a laser light delivered along fibreoptic cables. When the laser is used on the skin the light must be absorbed by the tissue for clinical effect. Chromophores (e.g. water, melanin, haemoglobin or tattoo ink) are specifically targeted by laser light of certain wavelengths causing photothermal damage.

Vascular lesions can be treated with pulse dye laser (510 nanometer wavelength), KTP laser (585–595 nm) and ND:YAG (long pulse 1320 nm). Pigmented lesions such as benign epidermal and dermal pigmented lesions can be treated where the chromophore is melanin (e.g. ND:YAG 532–1064 nm). Tattoos can also be removed with various lasers to remove colours including black, blue, green and red pigments. Laser resurfacing has become more popular with pulsed CO_2 and erbium:YAG lasers for photodamaged facial skin and scars.

Potential problems with lasers include discomfort, pigmentation, scarring and infections for the patient (e.g. herpes simplex virus) and operator (e.g. human papilloma virus and HIV).

Xanthelasma treatment

95% trichloroacetic acid can be painted onto the xanthelasma. There is a risk of this acid entering the eye and so it is applied with a cotton bud or orange stick to ensure only the area involved is treated. Repeated treatments are often necessary.

Other options for xanthelasma treatment include curettage and cautery under local anaesthetic.

Botulinum toxin

This is used commonly for hyperhidrosis particularly in the axillary area. This can be a painful treatment but if high amounts of sweat are being produced it can be very effective. Multiple injections are required around the site affected (e.g. axilla, scalp) (Figure 9.3).

Nail surgery

Nail surgery may be required to take biopsies of pigmented lesions and other tumours of the nail matrix and nail bed. This requires prior ring block and haemostasis is important. Special nail instruments are required to elevate the nail and to expose the nail matrix and nail bed. The centre of the lesion should be biopsied and a punch or small incisional biopsy may be sufficient for histological diagnosis (Figure 9.4).

Mohs' micrographic surgery

This is a method invented by Mohs in the USA to completely remove invasive BCC under histological control. The initial bulk of the tumour is removed by curettage creating a saucer-like defect. A further margin of skin is removed from the side and base of the wound and a horizontal section is taken of the surgical margin. The entire surgical margin can be examined histologically and then correlated to the area that may need further skin margins removed (Figure 9.5).

Mohs' surgery is useful for excision of BCC and SCC on the face where skin preservation is important (e.g. eyelids and nose). This is the treatment of choice for undefined margins or morphoeic BCC. It is time consuming and expensive and requires great surgical expertise to ensure good results.

Closure may require full thickness skin grafts, skin flap repairs or secondary intention healing.

Key points

- Laser treatments are widely available; however, the appropriate laser needs to be determined by the type of lesion to be treated.
- Mohs' surgery is a very specialised technique used to remove ill-defined tumours at critical sites.

▶ **Warning**

Liquid nitrogen cryotherapy is quick and easy to use but can leave disfiguring pigmentary changes and scarring.

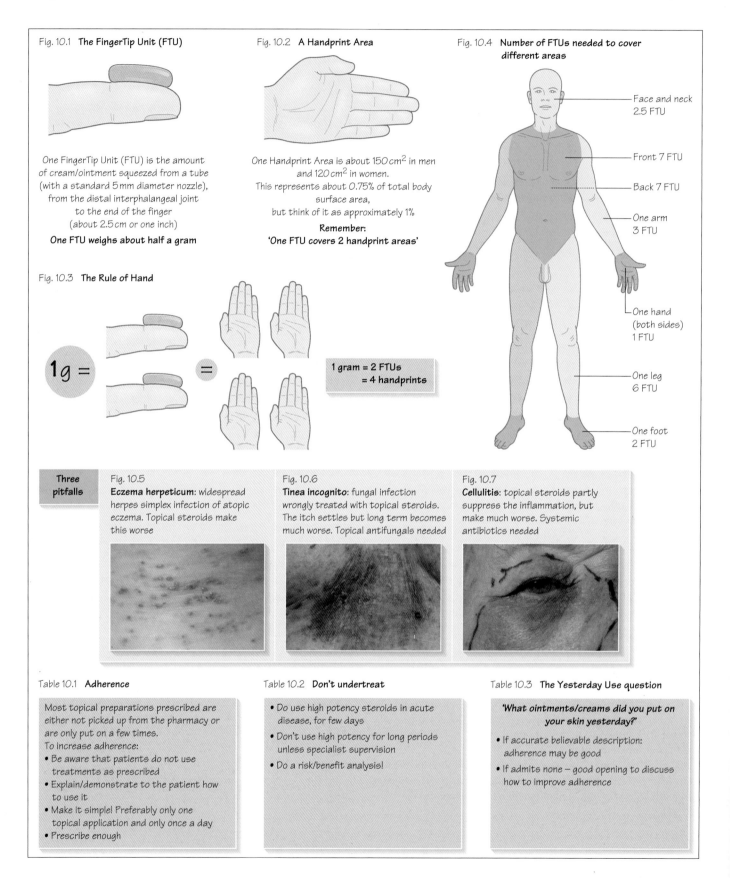

Fig. 10.1 **The FingerTip Unit (FTU)**

One FingerTip Unit (FTU) is the amount of cream/ointment squeezed from a tube (with a standard 5mm diameter nozzle), from the distal interphalangeal joint to the end of the finger (about 2.5cm or one inch)

One FTU weighs about half a gram

Fig. 10.2 **A Handprint Area**

One Handprint Area is about 150 cm² in men and 120 cm² in women. This represents about 0.75% of total body surface area, but think of it as approximately 1%

Remember:
'One FTU covers 2 handprint areas'

Fig. 10.4 **Number of FTUs needed to cover different areas**

Face and neck 2.5 FTU
Front 7 FTU
Back 7 FTU
One arm 3 FTU
One hand (both sides) 1 FTU
One leg 6 FTU
One foot 2 FTU

Fig. 10.3 **The Rule of Hand**

1g = = 1 gram = 2 FTUs = 4 handprints

Three pitfalls

Fig. 10.5 **Eczema herpeticum**: widespread herpes simplex infection of atopic eczema. Topical steroids make this worse

Fig. 10.6 **Tinea incognito**: fungal infection wrongly treated with topical steroids. The itch settles but long term becomes much worse. Topical antifungals needed

Fig. 10.7 **Cellulitis**: topical steroids partly suppress the inflammation, but make much worse. Systemic antibiotics needed

Table 10.1 **Adherence**

Most topical preparations prescribed are either not picked up from the pharmacy or are only put on a few times.
To increase adherence:
• Be aware that patients do not use treatments as prescribed
• Explain/demonstrate to the patient how to use it
• Make it simple! Preferably only one topical application and only once a day
• Prescribe enough

Table 10.2 **Don't undertreat**

• Do use high potency steroids in acute disease, for few days
• Don't use high potency for long periods unless specialist supervision
• Do a risk/benefit analysis!

Table 10.3 **The Yesterday Use question**

'What ointments/creams did you put on your skin yesterday?'

• If accurate believable description: adherence may be good
• If admits none – good opening to discuss how to improve adherence

Dermatology at a Glance, First Edition. Mahbub M.U. Chowdhury, Ruwani P. Katugampola, and Andrew Y. Finlay.

Topical skin treatment has a huge advantage over systemic therapy. The drug can go direct to the part of the skin that is diseased so high concentrations can be used with minimal risk. Cardiac drugs can harm the skin, but topical skin drugs do not harm the heart!

What influences absorption?

- Body site: the palm has very thick stratum corneum so absorbs little. The scrotum has thin stratum corneum so absorbs a great deal.
- Stratum corneum function: if the stratum corneum is moist (e.g. in body folds) much more will be absorbed than in dry exposed areas.
- Influence of the disease: if the stratum corneum is lost or diseased absorption is easier. So in treating psoriasis the drug gets in more easily at the diseased sites than the surrounding normal skin.
- Size of what is being absorbed: if the molecule is too large, very little will get in. Penetration enhancers such as propylene glycol may be added to topical drugs to increase drug absorption.
- Most topical drugs never get into the skin but end up on clothes.
- All topical drugs that get into the skin are eventually absorbed into the circulation, but the quantity is usually very small.

What is a cream?

A cream is a semi-solid mixture of water and lipids. Creams usually look opaque white (like fresh cream). Water and lipids do not blend, but can form an 'emulsion' in which small droplets of one are suspended in the other: either droplets of lipids in water or droplets of water in lipids. If the cream is 'lipids in water' (e.g. aqueous cream), it will evaporate and so is cooling, and the cream will mix with water so it can be washed off. If the cream is 'water in lipids' (e.g. oily cream), it is more difficult to wash off. Because creams contain water, they can spread easily over moist areas of diseased skin whereas ointments slip off.

What is in a cream?

- Active drug
- Base (the mixture of water and lipids)
- Emulsifying agents (which help to stabilise the emulsion)
- Antibacterials
- Perfumes (sometimes)

There may be a risk of developing allergic contact dermatitis to these different components, even though the active drug is not allergenic.

What is an ointment?

Ointments are semi-solid mixtures of lipids (no water). They feel greasy and look transparent and grey. Drugs such as corticosteroids may be added to both cream and ointment bases.

Ointments stick well to dry diseased skin.

'If it's dry, use an ointment, if it's wet, use a cream.'

What is a lotion?

A lotion is a liquid, usually water or sometimes alcohol, containing a medication. The liquid evaporates, leaving the medication spread over the surface.

What is an emollient?

An emollient (or 'moisturiser') is something that moisturises and softens the skin surface. Both creams and ointments can be emollients.

How often should drugs be applied?

The pharmaco-kinetics of many commonly used topical drugs are not well worked out. Traditionally, topical drugs have been used 2–3 times per day, often with no real evidence. There may sometimes be a patient-perceived benefit from the emollient action of some drugs, encouraging more frequent use than is pharmacologically necessary. Probably potent topical steroids would be equally effective used only once daily. Adherence is greater for once daily than for twice daily.

Topical steroids

Topical steroids revolutionised treatment of inflammatory skin disease in the 1950s. They are still the first choice for most inflammatory skin conditions.

The myths: 'Topical steroids are dangerous.' 'They should only ever be used very sparingly.'

The facts: Topical steroids have a range of potencies (strengths):
- *Mild potency:* minimal risk of side-effects. Least effective. e.g. hydrocortisone 0.5%, 1.0%, 2.5%.
- *Moderate potency:* minimal risk of side-effects. Mildly effective. e.g. clobetasone butyrate (Eumovate®).
- *Strong potency:* side-effects only if used daily for >2–3 weeks. Safe to use for few days in acute situations. Very effective. e.g. betamethasone valerate (Betnovate®).
- *Very strong potency:* high risk of side-effects. Extremely effective. e.g. clobetasol propionate (Dermovate®). Needed for resistant conditions (e.g. discoid lupus erythematosus), poor absorption sites (e.g. palms).

Side effects of potent topical steroids if used widely in the long term

Skin:
- Thinning of dermis: 'atrophy'
- Telangiectasia
- Rosacea, acne, peri-oral dermatitis
- Hirsutism
- Fragility of skin, easy bruising and tearing
- Contact allergy (see Chapter 30).

Systemic absorption (inflamed skin absorbs drugs more easily):
- Cushing's syndrome.

Topical tacrolimus and pimecrolimus

- Anti-inflammatory but not corticosteroids
- No skin thinning
- Local immunosuppressants
- Concern about long-term potential (so far unproven) for increasing skin cancer in sun exposed sites treated.

Key points

- Very inflamed skin is disabling and uncomfortable.
- Potent steroids have minimal risks used in the short term.
- A FingerTip Unit weighs 0.5 g and spreads over two handprints.

► **Warning**

Treatment often fails because of poor adherence.

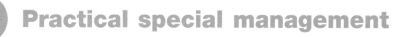

11 Practical special management

Table 11.1

Examples of dermatology day care services

- Patient education on application of topical treatments e.g. eczema
- Intensive topical treatments e.g. for psoriasis, eczema
- Regular review and monitoring of patients with 'unstable' inflammatory skin diseases e.g. eczema
- Phototherapy (Chapter 39)
- Management of leg ulcers (Chapter 45)
- Post-operative wound care following skin surgery e.g. following skin graft, suture removal
- Infusion and monitoring of patients on biological therapy for severe psoriasis
- Iontophoresis for palmar plantar hyperhidrosis

Table 11.2

Skin conditions treated with radiotherapy

Benign lesions	Malignant lesions
• Keloid scars	• Basal cell carcinoma • Squamous cell carcinoma • Cutaneous lymphomas (T and B cell sub-types) • Kaposi's sarcoma • Angiosarcoma • Merkel cell carcinoma

Table 11.3 **Potential complications of radiotherapy**

Acute complications	Long-term complications
• Redness (erythema) • Peeling (desquamation) of the skin on treated area • Mild bleeding	• Skin atrophy with telangiectasia • Fibrosis of skin • Hyper or hypo-pigmentation of the skin • Alopecia of treated site (e.g. scalp) • Skin malignancies at site of radiotherapy (e.g. squamous cell carcinoma)

Fig. 11.1 **Application of moisturisers**

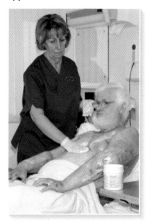

Fig. 11.2 **Application of coal tar**

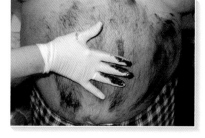

Fig. 11.5 **Infliximab infusion for severe psoriasis**

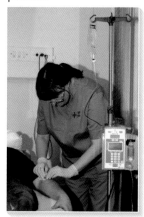

Fig 11.6 **Iontophoresis of the** (a) **hands and** (b) **feet**

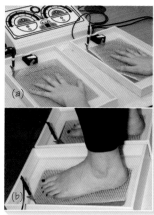

Fig. 11.3 (a) **Dithranol**
(b) **application of dithranol**

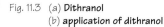
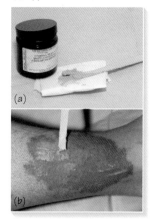

Fig. 11.4 **Zinc impregnated bandaging**
(a) either moisturisers or topical corticosteroids applied to the skin,
(b) followed by the zinc impregnated bandages,
(c) followed by cotton bandages (e.g. Tubifast®) to hold things in place

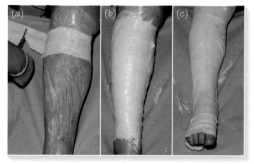

Fig. 11.7 **Application of topical cantharidin to a viral wart**

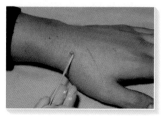

Dermatology at a Glance, First Edition. Mahbub M.U. Chowdhury, Ruwani P. Katugampola, and Andrew Y. Finlay.

Dermatology day care services

Dermatology care in the UK is primarily an outpatient service. In addition to the outpatient consultations, many patients benefit from dermatology day care services that are mainly nurse-led (Table 11.1). The following are examples of the services provided by a dermatology day care unit.

Patient education

Treatment of chronic inflammatory skin diseases such as eczema and psoriasis requires the use of several topical treatments including moisturisers and active treatments such as topical corticosteroids or calcineurin inhibitors.

Educating patients and parents of affected children regarding the appropriate application of the topical treatments, including quantities, when and how to use them, helps to improve treatment compliance. Patients also require education about self-administration of biological therapies for severe psoriasis.

Intensive topical treatment

Reasons for receiving topical treatment in a dermatology day care unit include the following:
• Severe extensive skin disease (e.g. eczema, psoriasis)
• Elderly individuals unable to reach body sites to apply treatment
• Co-morbidities that limit ability to use topical treatment (e.g. arthritis, impaired vision)
• Too messy to use at home (e.g. crude coal tar for psoriasis)
• Need careful application, as contact with unaffected skin may cause severe skin irritation (e.g. dithranol for large plaque psoriasis).

Moisturisers come in a variety of consistencies from lotions, creams to greasy emollients which can be used for any dry skin condition (e.g. eczema; Figure 11.1).

Coal tar, ranging in strength (1–20%), has been used for many years in the treatment of psoriasis and, less commonly, eczema (Figure 11.2). It is a relatively cheap, non-toxic treatment. Its exact mechanism of action is not known, but is thought to have anti-pruritic, anti-microbial and anti-inflammatory properties. Because of its thick black consistency and smell, treatment in patients' own homes is not practical or acceptable, and therefore requires day treatment. Coal tar is applied to the affected skin, then covered with light cotton bandages and washed away after 2 hours. Treatment is repeated on a daily basis, with increasing strength of coal tar, until disease clearance.

Dithranol (anthralin), ranging in strength (0.1–10%), has also been used for many years as a successful treatment for plaque psoriasis (Figure 11.3a,b). Its exact mechanism of action is not known. It stains and irritates unaffected skin. Dithranol is carefully applied only to the psoriatic plaques, the areas covered with light cotton bandages and left for 30–60 minutes (short contact therapy). It is then removed with cotton wool and the skin washed. Treatment is repeated daily, with increasing strength of dithranol, until disease clearance.

Bandaging is used in the treatment of inflammatory skin diseases affecting limbs. During treatment with coal tar or dithranol, light cotton bandages (e.g. Tubinet®) are used for occlusion. Light cotton bandages are also used over moisturisers or topical corticosteroids to contain the treatment on the skin, increase absorption and prevent direct trauma to the skin from scratching. Zinc impregnated bandages are effective for the treatment of atopic eczema and nodular prurigo (Figure 11.4a–c).

Other treatments undertaken in dermatology day units

Phototherapy See Chapter 39.

Biological therapy One of the biological therapies for severe psoriasis, infliximab, requires intravenous infusions at set time intervals and monitoring of the patient during infusions for adverse drug reactions (Figure 11.5).

Iontophoresis Excessive sweating (hyperhidrosis) of the palms and/or soles can be treated with a course of iontophoresis. This involves passing a small electric current while the affected hands and/or feet are immersed in a shallow bowl of tap water (Figure 11.6a,b), sometimes with glycopyrronium bromide.

Cantharidin treatment This is a toxic chemical produced by beetles. Its dilute form is used to treat viral warts that have not responded to conventional treatments (e.g. topical salicylic acid, cryotherapy). As blistering follows application, the treatment should be applied by an experienced nurse (Figure 11.7).

Management of leg ulcers This is discussed in Chapter 45. In some hospitals, leg ulcers are managed by dedicated wound care services, while in others ulcers are managed in dermatology day care units.

Radiotherapy

Radiotherapy is occasionally used for skin malignancies as either definite, adjuvant post-surgical or palliative treatment (Table 11.2). It utilises ionising electromagnetic radiation to damage rapidly dividing tumour DNA. Surrounding normal tissue can also be affected, resulting in potential complications (Table 11.3). Damage to normal tissue is reduced by treating with small divided doses (fractions) of radiation. It is the primary treatment option for skin malignancies in patients unsuitable for surgery (very elderly with multiple co-morbidities) and/or patient preference. It is also used as adjuvant therapy for peri-neural invasion or lymph node metastases associated with surgically excised squamous cell carcinomas.

Key points

• Dermatology day care services have an important role in education, treatment and monitoring of patients with a wide range of dermatological diseases.
• Radiotherapy is a non-surgical treatment option for management of skin malignancies.

► **Warning**

A long-term complication of radiotherapy is development of skin malignancies such as squamous cell carcinomas.

12 Psoriasis

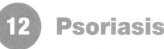

Table 12.1
Systemic treatments and side effects

PUVA and UVB	Burning, skin cancer
Methotrexate	Marrow suppression, indigestion, liver damage
Ciclosporin	Hypertension, renal damage, skin cancer
Acitretin	Teratogenic, dry lips, hyperlipidaemia
Mycophenolate mofetil	Gastro-intestinal upset, leukopenia
Biologics	Immune suppression, tuberculosis reactivation

Table 12.2
How to measure psoriasis, to inform decisions and monitor progress

- **Handprint:** 1% of body surface area (see Chapter 10)
- **PASI:** measures redness, scaling, thickness and area over four body regions. Score range 0–72, but most patients' scores are <10
- **DLQI:** used to assess how badly the patient's life is being affected (see Chapter 5)
- **The Rule of Tens:** If the Body Surface Area >10%, or the PASI >10 or the DLQI >10, this means that the psoriasis is 'severe'. Active therapy, possibly systemic, is required

Fig. 12.1
Guttate psoriasis: multiple small lesions

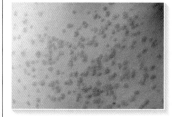

Fig. 12.2
Typical plaque psoriasis

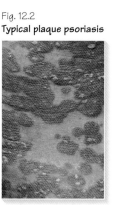

Fig. 12.3
Very widespread plaques over back of child

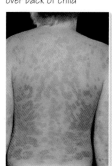

Fig. 12.4
Typical sites of psoriasis

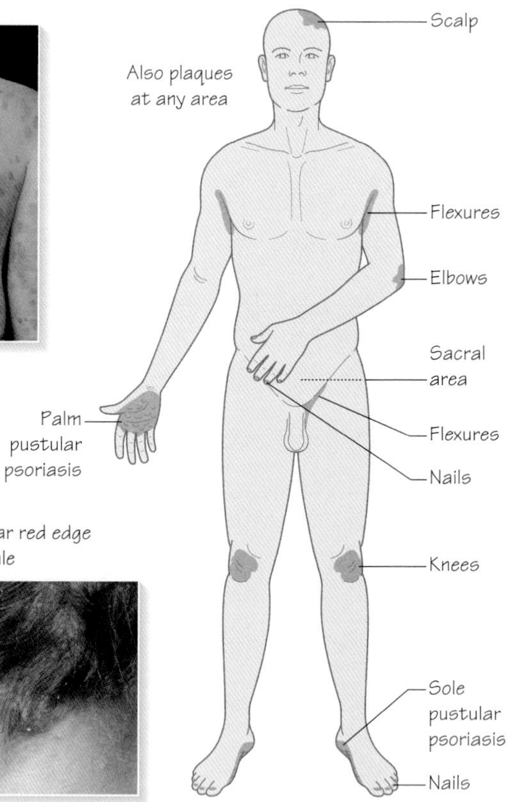

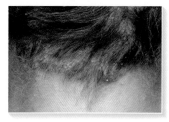

Scalp
Also plaques at any area
Flexures
Elbows
Sacral area
Palm pustular psoriasis
Flexures
Nails
Knees
Sole pustular psoriasis
Nails

Fig. 12.5
Flexural psoriasis: symmetrical shiny red areas with minimal scale in perianal area

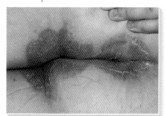

Fig. 12.6
Yellow separation (onycholysis) and pitting of nail

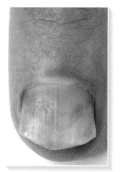

Fig. 12.7
Scalp psoriasis: clear red edge and much silvery scale

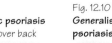

Fig. 12.8
Scalp psoriasis showing scale adherent to hairs – pityriasis amiantacea (don't confuse with nits)

Fig. 12.9
Erythrodermic psoriasis – widespread over back

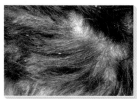

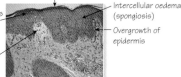

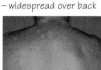

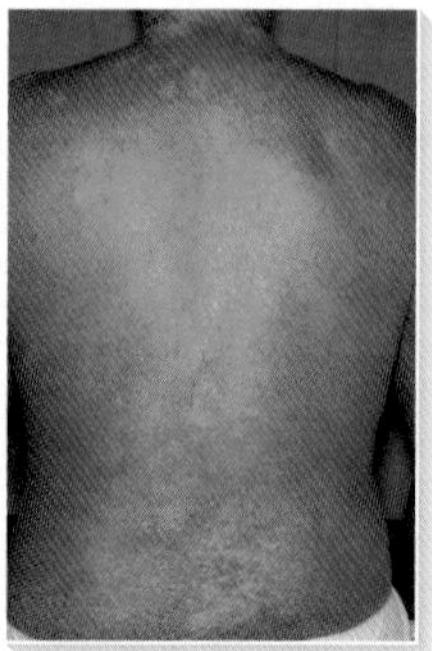

Fig. 12.10
Generalised pustular psoriasis involving shin

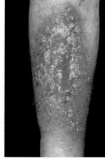

Fig. 12.11
Palmoplantar pustulosis – typical pustules on palm

Fig. 12.12 **Histology of psoriasis**

Thickening of stratum corneum, containing immature keratinocytes still containing nuclei (parakeratosis)
White blood cells in epidermis forming abscesses (Munro microabscesses)
Oedema and dilated blood vessels in dermal papillae
Intercellular oedema (spongiosis)
Overgrowth of epidermis

Dermatology at a Glance, First Edition. Mahbub M.U. Chowdhury, Ruwani P. Katugampola, and Andrew Y. Finlay.

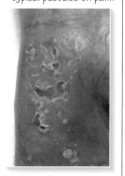

Clinical presentations

Psoriasis can start at any age, although the most common times are in the teens and in the forties and fifties. There is often a family history. About 3% of people develop psoriasis at some time in their lives. Children may present with 'guttate' (drop-like) psoriasis (Figure 12.1), multiple small red scaly areas, a few days after streptococcal throat infection.

There are multiple areas of red, slightly raised and scaly skin 'plaques' (Figures 12.2 and 12.3). Plaques have a clear edge and are often symmetrical. If scratched, they bleed more easily than normal skin. Knees, elbows and scalp are often affected, but all areas can be involved (Figure 12.4). Lesions last many months or years, may slowly enlarge and coalesce and can be itchy. Patients are most concerned by the appearance, the scales and the huge impact that the disease can have on their lives.

When the groin, axillae or other body folds are affected, the scale comes off easily in these moist areas so there is a shiny red appearance (Figure 12.5). Often, the fingernails are affected, with multiple small pits, discoloration and thickening (Figure 12.6). Toenails are also affected and can look like fungal infection.

Scalp psoriasis (Figures 12.7 and 12.8) can be felt better than seen, although if you part the hair, you see grey matted scale instead of normal scalp skin. Scalp psoriasis has a clear edge, typically with some areas unaffected, in contrast to dandruff that affects the whole scalp.

Rarely, the psoriasis becomes very extensive, with most of the skin becoming red and scaly (erythrodermic, Figure 12.9). This leads to:
• Increased fluid loss through the skin
• Increased protein loss
• Mild heart failure, as 25% of the cardiac output may be diverted to the skin
• Although the skin feels hot, there is great heat loss from radiation, resulting in hypothermia.

Very rarely, all areas can become covered by sterile pustules (Figure 12.10). This dermatology emergency, acute generalised pustular psoriasis, should not be confused with chronic localised palmoplantar pustulosis (Figure 12.11) that only affects palms and soles in smokers.

Co-morbidities

Psoriatic arthritis affects 30% of patients. There are 5 types: single large joint arthritis, distal interphalangeal arthritis, arthritis similar to rheumatoid but less severe, arthritis mutilans of fingers and toes, and spondylitis and/or sacroiliitis.

People with severe psoriasis usually have other problems with their health. Co-morbidities include obesity, hypertension, cardiac problems, diabetes, hyperlipidaemia and alcohol dependence.

Pathogenesis

First, you need to have a genetic susceptibility: the *PSOR1* location on chromosome 9 and other genes controlling inflammatory mediators are likely culprits. Once the condition starts, an immune process occurs. T lymphocytes move out of the blood vessels in the skin into the dermis. These spark off the release of chemical messengers, cytokines such as tumour necrosis factor-alpha, which result in the skin becoming inflamed and the epidermis becoming thickened and producing many more keratinocytes than usual, hence the scaliness. Why this process happens in localised often symmetrical areas remains a mystery.

Diagnosis

The diagnosis is usually made clinically from the history and typical appearance. The histology shows massively thickened epidermis, increased thickness of the stratum corneum, increased blood vessels nearer the surface (hence the redness) and inflammation in the upper dermis (Figure 12.12).

Treatment

Topical treatment

Most people with psoriasis have only a few lesions. Keeping the scale under control is important and frequently applying emollients may be all that is needed. For more active therapy, topical calcipotriol (a vitamin D analogue) is simple to apply and not too messy. Topical corticosteroids can be used alone or in combination with calcipotriol. If they are used over wide areas or continuously over months, there may be localised dermal thinning or even problems from systemic absorption. Topical dithranol (anthralin) is seldom used because it stains the skin (and the clothes) and can cause irritation. However, it is very effective if used carefully. If day care dermatology nursing treatment is available, patients can be helped with their treatment and compliance may improve (see Chapter 11).

Ultraviolet treatment (see Chapter 39)

Widespread psoriasis can be treated with narrow-band UVB (ultraviolet B radiation, wavelength 311 nm) or with PUVA (oral or topical psoralens and ultraviolet A). Patients have to attend twice weekly for 8–10 weeks; they get a nice tan but the lifetime number of treatments has to be limited to reduce the risk of skin cancer.

Systemic treatment (Table 12.1)

If topical treatments or UV fails, or if the Rule of Tens (see Chapter 5) (Table 12.2) is reached, then systemic treatment is probably indicated, even though all systemic therapies have risks of side effects. Oral methotrexate, ciclosporin, acitretin and mycophenolate mofetil are the first line oral therapies. If these fail, then biologics are used, such as infliximab, etanercept, adalimumab or ustekinumab; they work by specifically targeting key inflammatory messengers. They are given by injection or intravenous infusion and are highly effective, but very expensive. As they are relatively new drugs, their long-term benefits and side effects are not yet known.

Obesity, hypertension, cardiac problems, diabetes and alcohol dependency should be searched for and treated in parallel.

Key points

• Match the aggressiveness of intervention to the impact of the disease on the patient's life.
• Compliance with therapy is very difficult in a chronic disease. Make treatment as simple as possible.

► **Warning**

Erythrodermic psoriasis needs urgent inpatient treatment.

Table 13.1 Diagnostic criteria for atopic dermatitis

Must have:
- Itchy skin in the last 12 months

Plus three or more of the following:
- History of flexural involvement
- History of asthma and/or hay fever (or in children <4 years, history of atopy in first degree relatives)
- History of a generally dry skin
- Visible flexural eczema
- Onset in the first two years of life

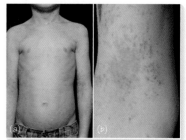

Fig. 13.1
Acute infantile atopic dermatitis on the face

Fig. 13.2
(a) Child with widespread acute atopic dermatitis and
(b) close-up of the typical erythematous papules at the antecubital fossa

Fig. 13.3
Atopic dermatitis of the face and upper trunk in an adult

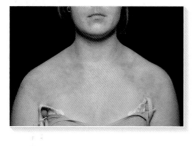

Fig. 13.4
(a) Chronic eczema of the legs and
(b) close-up of the lichenified plaques at the flexures

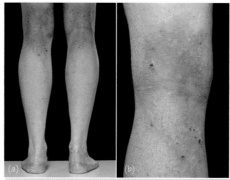

Fig. 13.6
Eczema herpeticum on the face

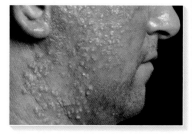

Fig. 13.7
Striae due to prolonged use of potent topical corticosteroids

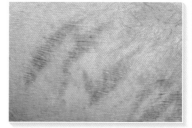

Fig. 13.5 The aetiology of atopic dermatitis

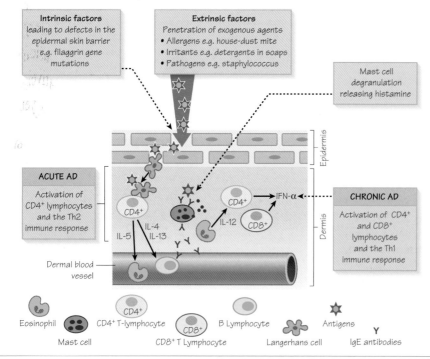

Intrinsic factors
leading to defects in the epidermal skin barrier e.g. filaggrin gene mutations

Extrinsic factors
Penetration of exogenous agents
- Allergens e.g. house-dust mite
- Irritants e.g. detergents in soaps
- Pathogens e.g. staphylococcus

Mast cell degranulation releasing histamine

ACUTE AD
Activation of CD4+ lymphocytes and the Th2 immune response

IL-5 IL-4 IL-13

Dermal blood vessel

Epidermis

Dermis

CD4+

CD4+

CD8+

IL-12

IFN-α

CHRONIC AD
Activation of CD4+ and CD8+ lymphocytes and the Th1 immune response

Eosinophil Mast cell CD4+ T-lymphocyte CD8+ T Lymphocyte B Lymphocyte Langerhans cell Antigens Y IgE antibodies

Table 13.2
Aims of management of atopic dermatitis

- Patient and parent education about the disease and its management
- Participation of patient and parent(s) in treatment of their AD
- Restore epidermal barrier function with emollients
- Control skin inflammation and maintenance in remission with topical corticosteroids and calcineurin inhibitors
- Consider second-line therapy for severe disease, e.g. phototherapy, systemic immunosuppressants
- Prevent exacerbations secondary to infection, irritants and allergens
- Maintain long-term disease control

Dermatology at a Glance, First Edition. Mahbub M.U. Chowdhury, Ruwani P. Katugampola, and Andrew Y. Finlay.

Atopy is the tendency to develop hypersensitivity to allergens as a result of genetic predisposition and environmental factors. Atopic diseases include atopic dermatitis (AD), hay fever and asthma. AD is a common, chronic, relapsing and remitting inflammatory skin disease; its prevalence is about 5–15% in children and 2–10% in adults. The diagnostic criteria for AD are summarised in Table 13.1.

Clinical patterns according to age

Infantile AD Onset is within the first 6 months and persists until the age of 2–3 years. Usually affects the head and neck (Figure 13.1).

Childhood AD Onset is within the first few years of life and persists until or into puberty. Typically affects flexures (e.g. antecubital and popliteal fossae, neck) (Figure 13.2).

Adult AD Onset is usually in those in their twenties or thirties. It can affect head and neck, flexures of limbs and trunk (Figure 13.3). There is often a previous history of infantile or childhood AD.

Clinical features (Figures 13.1–13.4)

• **Acute** (or acute on chronic) **AD** presents with itchy erythematous papules, patches and vesicles with or without erosions on the affected areas.
• **Chronic AD** appears as thickened dry skin with prominence of skin markings (lichenification), often with excoriations and post-inflammatory pigmentary changes (hyper- or hypopigmentation).

Aetiology and pathogenesis (Figure 13.5)

In normal skin, keratinocytes and intercellular lipids form the epidermal barrier which retains water and prevents the penetration of exogenous agents (e.g. allergens and irritants) into the skin. The aetiology of AD is multi-factorial, with genetic and environmental influences, epidermal barrier defects, penetration of exogenous agents into the skin and activation of the immune response.

Mutations in filaggrin genes have been linked to AD in about 10% of individuals with AD in Europe. Filaggrin is an epidermal skin barrier protein that has a role in the aggregation of the keratin cytoskeleton during epidermal differentiation.

In acute AD, the dermal Th2 immune response is activated by uptake and presentation of antigens by the epidermal dendritic antigen presenting cells (i.e. Langerhans cells) to CD4[+] lymphocytes in the dermis and blood vessels. These cells produce Th2 pro-inflammatory cytokines (e.g. interleukin [IL] 4, 5, 13) which recruit eosinophils, B lymphocytes and induce immunoglobulin E (IgE) production. IgE activates histamine release by mast cells leading to itching. In the chronic phase of AD, eosinophils release IL-12 activating the Th1 immune response leading to release of α-interferon (IFN-α) by CD4[+] and CD8[+] T lymphocytes.

Complications of atopic dermatitis

Bacterial infection The skin of AD patients is colonised with *Staphylococcus aureus*; their exotoxins act as superantigens which activate the inflammatory process in acute AD. *Staphylococcus* also causes superadded infection, leading to flare-ups of AD and impetigo (exudate, yellow crusting, blistering [bullous impetigo]).

Eczema herpeticum (see Chapter 19) is localised or widespread herpes simplex infection of skin affected by AD (Figure 13.6). It presents with grouped vesicles and/or pustules which progress to superficial erosions, crusting and heal without scarring. Ophthalmology review is essential when the face is involved.

Erythroderma See Chapter 16.

Allergic contact dermatitis including to the patient's own topical treatments (e.g. steroids and/or the preservatives) should be considered in those with treatment-resistant AD (see Chapter 30).

Management

• Patient education on the management of their AD.
• Regular moisturising breaks the itch–scratch cycle and prevents exacerbations. The choice of moisturiser(s) (see Chapter 10) is best decided with the patient to improve treatment compliance. Soap substitute emollients should be used instead of conventional soaps which dry the skin, leading to exacerbation of AD.
• Oral anti-histamines are useful for itch relief. Sedating anti-histamines such as chlorphenamine are useful at night.
• Topical corticosteroids are the treatment of choice for controlling the inflammation in AD. The lowest effective potency of topical steroids is used, depending on the patient's age and body site, and weaned off once clinical clearance has been achieved (see Chapter 10). Mild potencies are preferred for the face and flexures; moderate to high potencies for limited periods to other body sites.
• Complications of the long-term use of topical steroids include skin atrophy, striae (Figure 13.7), glaucoma and growth retardation in children resulting from suppression of the pituitary–adrenal axis.
• Topical calcineurin inhibitors (tacrolimus and pimecrolimus) are topical immunosuppressants used for maintenance of remission in AD, once the acute flares have been controlled with topical corticosteroids. Their advantage is the lack of steroid-associated complications. However, in view of their immunosuppressant effect, these treatments should not be used on infected eczema.
• Bandaging of limbs affected by AD is often used either with moisturisers, zinc or topical corticosteroids (see Chapter 11).
• Phototherapy (see Chapter 39) can be used for widespread AD resistant to topical treatment. Systemic steroids (oral prednisolone) for up to 2 weeks are occasionally used to control severe widespread AD. Systemic immunosuppressants (e.g. azathioprine, ciclosporin, mycophenolate mofetil) are useful in the long-term control of widespread severe AD unresponsive to the above topical treatments.
• Management of superadded infections includes swabbing affected areas for bacterial and viral cultures and prescribing antibiotics (e.g. flucloxacillin) and/or antiviral (e.g. aciclovir) therapy.

Key points

• Management of AD includes regular moisturising, control of acute flares with topical corticosteroids and maintaining remission with topical calcineurin inhibitors with avoidance of potential triggers.
• Possible causes for flare-ups of AD include poor treatment compliance, superadded infection or allergic contact dermatitis.

► **Warning**

Inappropriate long-term use of potent topical corticosteroids is associated with potential complications.

---

14 Acne and teenage skin

Table 14.1
Skin diseases that may affect teenagers

- **Inflammatory:** acne, eczema (see Chapter 13), psoriasis (see Chapter 12)
- **Infections:** pityriasis versicolor (see Chapter 20)
- **Autoimmune:** vitiligo (see Chapter 37), alopecia areata (see Chapter 25)
- **Benign skin lesions:** congenital or acquired naevi (see Chapter 33), viral warts (see Chapter 19)
- **Malignant skin lesions:** malignant melanoma (see Chapter 35)
- **Vascular lesions:** vascular malformation (see Chapter 26)
- **Self-induced:** dermatitis artefacta (see Chapter 44)

Table 14.2
Points to consider when consulting a teenager with a skin disease

- Impact of skin disease on psychological well being
- Impact of psychological issues on skin disease
- Impact of chronic disease and its treatment on education and social activities
- Impact of media and peer pressure to have 'perfect skin'
- Cosmetic issues regarding skin lesions/rashes
- Patient education/disease prevention
- Treatment compliance

Fig. 14.1 **Severe psoriasis of both palms** causing functional and psychological impact

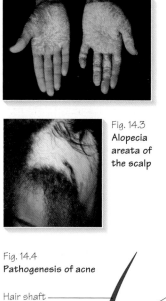

Fig. 14.2 **Vitiligo of the lower legs** – note the contrast between the depigmented patches of vitiligo with the darker unaffected skin

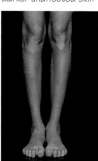

Fig. 14.3 **Alopecia areata of the scalp**

Fig. 14.5 **Open comedones and pustules**

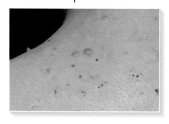

Fig. 14.6 **Inflammatory papules and pustules**

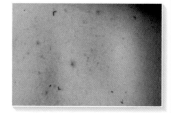

Fig. 14.4 **Pathogenesis of acne**

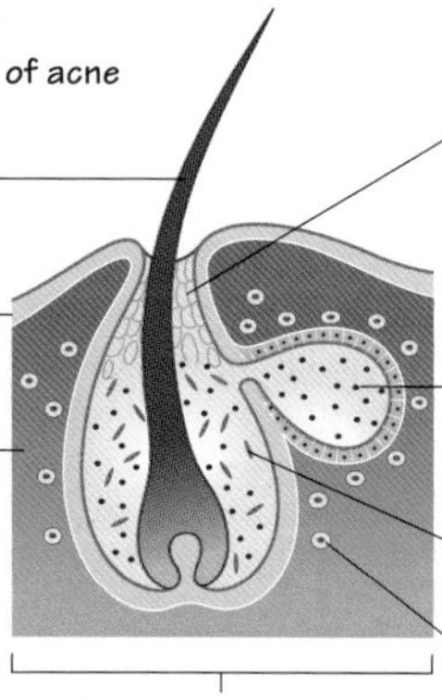

Hair shaft
Epidermis
Dermis
Hyperkeratinisation of infundibulum followed by shedding of keratinocytes into its lumen
Androgen-stimulated secretion of sebum by sebaceous glands
Proliferation of P. acnes
Dermal inflammation
Pilosebaceous unit

Fig. 14.7 **Severe nodular, cystic scarring acne**

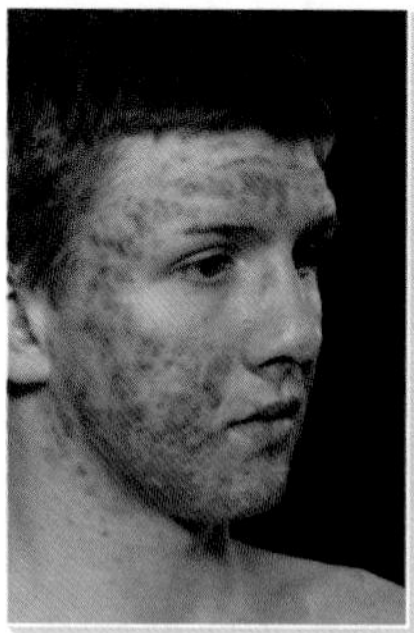

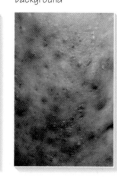

Fig. 14.8 **Close-up of severe acne** – note the comedones, pustules, nodules and scarring on an inflammatory background

Fig. 14.9 **Keloid scar formation following severe acne**

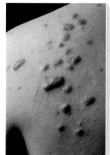

Table 14.3
Mode of action of acne treatments

Treatment	Mode of action
Topical retinoid	Reduction in epidermal hyperkeratinisation, anti-inflammatory
Topical benzoyl peroxide	Anti-inflammatory, anti-bacterial
Topical antibiotics	Anti-inflammatory, anti-bacterial
Oral antibiotics	Anti-inflammatory, anti-bacterial
Anti-androgen	Reduce sebaceous gland hyper-secretion
Oral isotretinoin	Reduce sebaceous gland hyper-secretion & epidermal hyperkeratinisation, anti-inflammatory

Dermatology at a Glance, First Edition. Mahbub M.U. Chowdhury, Ruwani P. Katugampola, and Andrew Y. Finlay.

Teenage years can be a stressful period during which many changes occur in the physical and psychological aspects of life. These issues should be borne in mind when consulting a teenager with any form of skin disease. Skin diseases that may affect teenagers are summarised in Table 14.1.

Points to consider when consulting a teenager with a skin disease (Table 14.2)

Skin diseases are often visible. This can impact on the psychological well-being of affected individuals, exacerbated by media and peer pressure to have 'perfect skin' (e.g. scarring acne, psoriasis, vitiligo or eczema affecting exposed skin) (Figures 14.1–14.3 and 14.7). Psychological stress from domestic or school issues or the skin disease itself may cause further flares (e.g. psoriasis).

Severe chronic skin diseases (e.g. psoriasis or eczema) may require frequent hospital appointments for day treatment, or inpatient therapy. These may disrupt educational and recreational activities.

Skin lesions on exposed skin may be cosmetically unacceptable for patients. Excision of benign lesions needs to be weighed against the cosmetic effect of the resulting scar. Cosmetic camouflage is beneficial for vitiligo or large vascular malformations.

Education is important in disease prevention and treatment compliance. For example, raising awareness of the skin cancer risk of sun beds, photo-protection measures and how to recognise a suspicious skin cancer. Similarly, developing a topical treatment regime practical and acceptable to the individual's daily routine can improve treatment compliance in chronic skin diseases.

Acne vulgaris

This is the most common skin disease affecting teenagers. It is associated with significant impact on psychological well-being. A disease of the pilosebaceous unit in the skin, pathogenesis of acne is multi-factorial (Fig 14.4) and includes the following:
• Hyperkeratinisation of the epidermis in the infundibulum of the hair follicles.
• Shedding and accumulation of keratinocytes within the lumen of the infundibulum.
• Stimulation of increased sebum production by androgen hormones.
• Proliferation of *Propionibacterium acnes*, a Gram-positive anaerobic bacterium, within the pilosebaceous units.
• Because of the narrow openings into the skin surface, the shed corneocytes, sebum and *P. acnes* accumulate within the pilosebaceous units which subsequently rupture.
• This leads to dermal inflammation, mainly consisting of neutrophils (early and late stages) and T-helper lymphocytes (late stages).
• Up-regulation of genes coding inflammatory cytokines including matrix metalloproteinases and interleukin-8.

Diagnosis is made clinically based on the types of lesions described below and the distribution of the rash characteristically affecting the face, back and shoulders to varying extents. Different stages of clinical severity exist, corresponding to the stages of pathogenesis described above:
• Comedones (Figure 14.5) are non-inflamed early lesions of acne. Closed comedones ('white-heads') are small, approximately 1–2 mm skin-coloured papules. Open comedones ('black-heads') are papules with a central keratin plug consisting of shed keratin. Comedones can lead to subtle ice-pick scars.
• Papules and pustules (Figure 14.6) develop with the onset of inflammation. These erythematous lesions often lead to scarring.
• Nodules and cysts are associated with marked inflammation and tenderness and lead to scarring (Figures 14.7 and 14.8).

Complications of acne include the following:
• Scarring ranging from subtle pitted ('ice-pick') to keloid scars (Figure 14.9).
• Psychological distress due to the disease itself and subsequent scarring.

The aim of treatment is disease control and prevention of scarring (Table 14.3). Choice of treatment(s) depends on the stage of clinical severity:
• *Mild comedones ± few papules:* topical benzoyl peroxide ± topical antibiotic (e.g. clindamycin), topical retinoid.
• *Moderately severe acne with papules and pustules with mild scarring:* the above topical treatment with a 3-month course of oral antibiotic (e.g. erythromycin, oxytetracycline, doxycycline). In female patients, an anti-androgen combined with oestrogen in the form of the oral contraceptive pill can be used (e.g. Dianette® containing 2 mg cyproterone acetate + 35 μg ethinylestradiol).
• *Severe acne with papules, pustules, nodules, cysts and scarring:* oral isotretinoin 0.5–1 mg/kg/day for 4–6 months. Isotretinoin is a retinoid and is teratogenic; therefore females of child-bearing age commenced on isotretinoin should be counselled and must use a reliable mode of contraception (e.g. oral contraceptive pill, intra-uterine contraceptive device).

In treatment resistant acne, consider possible underlying cause(s):
• Polycystic ovarian syndrome in females
• Ingestion or injection of anabolic steroids.

Key points

• Skin diseases can have a psychological impact in teenagers.
• Pathogenesis of acne is multi factorial and includes hyperkeratinisation, shedding and accumulation of keratinocytes within the pilosebacous unit, androgen-stimulated increased production of sebum and proliferation of *P. acnes* leading to dermal inflammation.
• Treatment of acne depends on disease severity.
• Treatment options include topical anti-bacterials with or without antibiotics, topical retinoids, oral antibiotics, anti-androgens (for females only) and oral isotretinoin.

► **Warning**

Females of child-bearing age with severe acne considered for oral isotretinoin should be counselled regarding its teratogenic effects. A reliable mode of contraception is needed 1 month prior to, during and 1 month post-treatment.

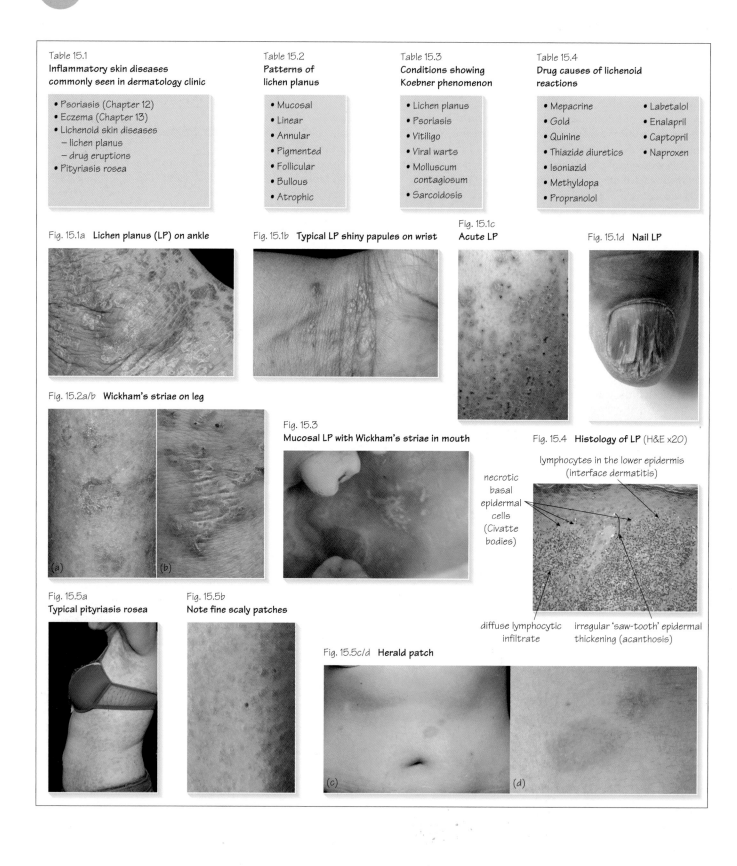

Table 15.1
Inflammatory skin diseases commonly seen in dermatology clinic

- Psoriasis (Chapter 12)
- Eczema (Chapter 13)
- Lichenoid skin diseases
  - lichen planus
  - drug eruptions
- Pityriasis rosea

Table 15.2
Patterns of lichen planus

- Mucosal
- Linear
- Annular
- Pigmented
- Follicular
- Bullous
- Atrophic

Table 15.3
Conditions showing Koebner phenomenon

- Lichen planus
- Psoriasis
- Vitiligo
- Viral warts
- Molluscum contagiosum
- Sarcoidosis

Table 15.4
Drug causes of lichenoid reactions

- Mepacrine
- Gold
- Quinine
- Thiazide diuretics
- Isoniazid
- Methyldopa
- Propranolol
- Labetalol
- Enalapril
- Captopril
- Naproxen

Fig. 15.1a   Lichen planus (LP) on ankle

Fig. 15.1b   Typical LP shiny papules on wrist

Fig. 15.1c
Acute LP

Fig. 15.1d   Nail LP

Fig. 15.2a/b   Wickham's striae on leg

(a)   (b)

Fig. 15.3
Mucosal LP with Wickham's striae in mouth

Fig. 15.4   Histology of LP (H&E x20)

lymphocytes in the lower epidermis (interface dermatitis)

necrotic basal epidermal cells (Civatte bodies)

diffuse lymphocytic infiltrate

irregular 'saw-tooth' epidermal thickening (acanthosis)

Fig. 15.5a
Typical pityriasis rosea

Fig. 15.5b
Note fine scaly patches

Fig. 15.5c/d   Herald patch

(c)   (d)

Dermatology at a Glance, First Edition. Mahbub M.U. Chowdhury, Ruwani P. Katugampola, and Andrew Y. Finlay.

Lichenoid disorders

'Lichenoid' can describe the appearance clinically of a shiny flat-topped papular rash or can suggest histology of band-like inflammatory cell infiltrate in the upper dermis with basal cell necrosis. Lichenoid eruptions can be due to a number of causes including lichen planus (LP), drug eruptions, graft versus host disease (GvHD) and pityriasis lichenoides (Table 15.1).

Lichen planus

Most people with cutaneous LP (>70%) have oral involvement; 10% present with this. LP is a T-cell mediated autoimmune inflammatory condition. There are possible genetic links and association with hepatitis C. LP presents as shiny, flat topped, violaceous polygonal papules on the skin (Figure 15.1). Papules vary in size and many clinical patterns are seen (Table 15.2). In typical presentations, with distribution on the dorsum of the ankles and wrists, a biopsy is not always required; however, LP can occur on any body site including the palms and soles.

Wickham's striae describes the surface white lines with a lace-like pattern (Figure 15.2). Hypertrophy and hyperpigmentation in darker skin types is common and linear lesions can occur along scratch marks or scars (Koebner's phenomenon) (Table 15.3). Itching is common but can be absent.

Mucosal areas (60%) in the mouth may cause pain and ulceration (Figure 15.3). Mucous membrane involvement may need patch testing to exclude allergy (e.g. mercury amalgam). The nails are affected (10%) with ridging (Figure 15.1d) and thinning of the nail plate and pterygium (adhesions between the posterior nailfold and nail plate). Scarring alopecia on the scalp with skin atrophy can cause permanent scarring.

Histopathology

Typical features are an irregular saw tooth thickening of the epidermis (acanthosis) with Civatte bodies (necrotic basal epidermal cells) and a lymphocytic inflammatory infiltrate (Figure 15.4). Specific features are seen in hypertrophic, atrophic, follicular and mucosal lichen planus. Differential diagnoses include plane warts, eczema and pityriasis rosea, and lichen simplex chronicus.

Prognosis and treatment

LP can clear spontaneously within a few weeks but most acute attacks will last for at least 6 months if untreated. Mucous membrane lesions may clear more slowly. Resolving lesions generally stop itching. Progression can occur with hypertrophy or hair loss if the scalp is affected.

Treatment is symptomatic and potent topical steroids (with occlusion) can be used to increase the absorption and effectiveness, particularly with hypertrophic LP. Generalised or LP unresponsive to topical treatments may require systemic therapy such as oral corticosteroids for short periods or retinoids (acitretin), ciclosporin or oral bath PUVA. Oral lesions may require betamethasone (Betnesol®) mouthwash or triamcinolone in Orabase®.

Other lichenoid reactions
Lichen planus-like eruption due to drugs

Many drugs are known to cause lichenoid and LP-like changes (Table 15.4). Mepacrine was used as an anti-malarial during the Second World War. Gold has been the most common recent drug causing LP-like eruptions, but this is now used less often for rheumatoid arthritis. Histologically, the pattern of lichenoid changes is similar to idiopathic LP. However, the presence of eosinophils may point more towards a drug reaction. Quinine and thiazide diuretics can cause a lichenoid photodermatitis which can appear more psoriasis-like. Hyperpigmentation and hair loss may be severe.

Previously, 25% of people using photographic colour developers developed acute eczematous and subacute lichenoid changes but automated equipment now minimises this risk.

Graft versus host disease

Skin manifestations are prominent in GvHD and can mimic LP. Bone marrow transplantation for severe haematological disorders including acute leukaemias may precipitate GvHD. This is due to lymphoid cells from an immunocompetent donor being introduced into an incompatible recipient who is then incapable of rejecting the lymphoid cells. The threat of GvHD is increased when the genotypes of the donor and recipient are not identical. The reaction varies from mild to severe, with over 70% mortality.

The process may be acute or chronic and most patients with GvHD have skin involvement. This presents 1 week to 3 months after transplantation (acute) or after 3 months (chronic). Patients with GvHD present with fever and erythema of the face, palms and soles with a generalised papular eruption. Differentials include drug reactions and infections. Chronic GvHD involves the skin, liver, upper respiratory and gastrointestinal tract. Local or general changes in the skin occur with sclerosis, ulceration, lichenoid changes, and hyper- or hypopigmentation with severe poikiloderma. Treatment for skin GvHD includes ciclosporin and phototherapy.

Pityriasis rosea

Pityriasis rosea is a common acute self-limiting disease affecting children and young adults. After being unwell, a typical 'herald patch' follows which is a large, 2–5 cm, inflamed well-defined scaly patch. A general eruption with new oval, pink to red fine scaly patches occurs 1–2 weeks later with collarette of scale surrounding the edge (Figure 15.5). These lesions can occur in a Christmas tree pattern occurring mainly on the trunk, neck and upper third of the arms and legs. The skin eruption fades within 3–6 weeks and can usually be diagnosed from the typical history and herald patch. Differentials include seborrhoeic dermatitis, drug eruption, secondary syphilis, urticaria and guttate psoriasis. Only minimal treatment is needed with topical emollients, mild to moderate strength topical steroids and, if not responsive, UVB.

Key points

- Lichen planus has many clinical patterns including mucosal.
- Lichenoid drug reactions can mimic lichen planus.
- Pityriasis rosea is an acute self-limiting disease in children and young adults.

▶ **Warning**

Graft versus host disease should be considered in any lichenoid skin eruption in severe haematological conditions.

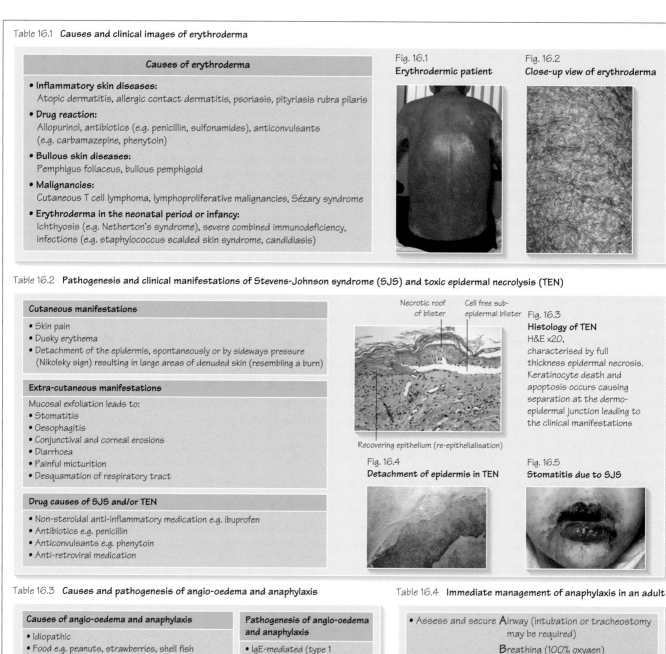

Table 16.1 Causes and clinical images of erythroderma

Causes of erythroderma

- **Inflammatory skin diseases:**
  Atopic dermatitis, allergic contact dermatitis, psoriasis, pityriasis rubra pilaris
- **Drug reaction:**
  Allopurinol, antibiotics (e.g. penicillin, sulfonamides), anticonvulsants (e.g. carbamazepine, phenytoin)
- **Bullous skin diseases:**
  Pemphigus foliaceus, bullous pemphigoid
- **Malignancies:**
  Cutaneous T cell lymphoma, lymphoproliferative malignancies, Sézary syndrome
- **Erythroderma in the neonatal period or infancy:**
  Ichthyosis (e.g. Netherton's syndrome), severe combined immunodeficiency, infections (e.g. staphylococcus scalded skin syndrome, candidiasis)

Fig. 16.1
Erythrodermic patient

Fig. 16.2
Close-up view of erythroderma

Table 16.2 Pathogenesis and clinical manifestations of Stevens-Johnson syndrome (SJS) and toxic epidermal necrolysis (TEN)

Cutaneous manifestations

- Skin pain
- Dusky erythema
- Detachment of the epidermis, spontaneously or by sideways pressure (Nikolsky sign) resulting in large areas of denuded skin (resembling a burn)

Extra-cutaneous manifestations

Mucosal exfoliation leads to:
- Stomatitis
- Oesophagitis
- Conjunctival and corneal erosions
- Diarrhoea
- Painful micturition
- Desquamation of respiratory tract

Drug causes of SJS and/or TEN

- Non-steroidal anti-inflammatory medication e.g. ibuprofen
- Antibiotics e.g. penicillin
- Anticonvulsants e.g. phenytoin
- Anti-retroviral medication

Necrotic roof of blister   Cell free sub-epidermal blister   Fig. 16.3
Histology of TEN
H&E x20, characterised by full thickness epidermal necrosis. Keratinocyte death and apoptosis occurs causing separation at the dermo-epidermal junction leading to the clinical manifestations

Recovering epithelium (re-epithelialisation)

Fig. 16.4
Detachment of epidermis in TEN

Fig. 16.5
Stomatitis due to SJS

Table 16.3 Causes and pathogenesis of angio-oedema and anaphylaxis

Causes of angio-oedema and anaphylaxis

- Idiopathic
- Food e.g. peanuts, strawberries, shell fish
- Latex
- Hereditary C1 esterase inhibitor deficiency (autosomal dominant)
- Medication, e.g. non-steroidal anti-inflammatories, aspirin, antibiotics, ACE inhibitors
- Contrast medium
- Bee or wasp sting

Pathogenesis of angio-oedema and anaphylaxis

- IgE-mediated (type 1 hypersensitivity) e.g. latex and food allergies
- Complement-mediated e.g. C1 esterase inhibitor deficiency

Release of vasodilator substances such as histamine +/– activation of the complement pathway leading to swelling of dermis and subcutaneous tissue

Fig. 16.6
Angio-oedema of the lips

Table 16.4 Immediate management of anaphylaxis in an adult

- Assess and secure Airway (intubation or tracheostomy may be required)
  Breathing (100% oxygen)
  Circulation (elevate legs, intravenous fluid if hypotensive)
- Commence cardiopulmonary resuscitation if appropriate

- Intramuscular adrenaline 500 mcg (0.5 ml of 1 in 1000) repeated every 5 minutes if required
- Intravenous hydrocortisone 200 mg
- Intravenous chlorphenamine 10 mg

Dermatology at a Glance, First Edition. Mahbub M.U. Chowdhury, Ruwani P. Katugampola, and Andrew Y. Finlay.

Erythroderma

Erythroderma is characterised by generalised erythema, scaling and exfoliation of the skin affecting at least 90% of the body surface area (Figures 16.1 and 16.2). It has many different causes (Table 16.1). The cause may not be identified in 20–30% of cases (idiopathic).

Complications occur due to skin failure and loss of skin function:
- Skin infections and septicaemia (loss of skin barrier function)
- Hypothermia (loss of thermoregulation)
- Peripheral oedema (loss of albumin)
- Tachycardia and high-output cardiac failure
- Renal failure (loss of fluid and electrolytes).

Management
- Identify and treat or withdraw underlying cause (e.g. drugs)
- Supportive care
- Prevention of complications.

The patient should be managed in a warm environment to prevent hypothermia, with regular monitoring of core body temperature, blood pressure, pulse, fluid balance and for evidence of sepsis.

Treatment:
- Fluid and electrolyte replacement, nutritional support
- Sedating anti-histamines for itching
- Frequent topical application of emollients
- Systemic antibiotics if evidence of infection
- Systemic steroids (oral prednisolone) may be considered if the underlying cause is likely to be drug induced.

Erythema multiforme

See Chapter 41.

Stevens–Johnson syndrome and toxic epidermal necrolysis

This is a disease spectrum, usually drug induced and characterised by potentially life-threatening muco-cutaneous exfoliation (Table 16.2; Figures 16.3–16.5). Stevens–Johnson syndrome (SJS) and toxic epidermal necrolysis (TEN) are defined by the affected body surface area (<10% = SJS, 10–30% = SJS–TEN overlap, >30% = TEN).

Complications are similar to that of erythroderma. Early diagnosis and management is vital to reduce mortality. SCORTEN is a scoring system used to predict mortality of patients with TEN. This includes indices such as patient's age, co-morbidities and laboratory markers (e.g. serum creatinine).

Management
Principles of management are similar to that of erythroderma. Use of systemic steroids is controversial because of increased risk of sepsis. Intravenous immunoglobulins may improve prognosis in TEN.

Angio-oedema and anaphylaxis

Different causes can lead to angio-oedema and anaphylaxis by release of vasodilator substances that result in swelling of dermis and subcutaneous tissue (Table 16.3). Angio-oedema is characterised by painless swelling of the skin, commonly the hands, eyelids, tongue and lips (Figure 16.6). Urticaria may or may not be present (see Chapter 32). Mucosal involvement can lead to life-threatening swelling of the upper airways and throat resulting in difficulty swallowing and breathing (anaphylaxis).

Management
- A detailed history to identify the potential cause(s).
- Further investigations may be indicated to identify the causative agent. If IgE-mediated reaction to latex or food is suspected, blood tests for serum IgE and allergen-specific RAST (radioallergosorbent test). If this test is negative, prick-testing should be considered, where full resuscitation is available (see Chapter 30). C1 esterase inhibitor, complement C3 and C4 levels should be measured when C1 esterase inhibitor deficiency is suspected.
- Angio-oedema is treated with a short course of oral steroids and H1 anti-histamines. In hereditary angio-oedema resulting from C1 esterase inhibitor deficiency, C1 inhibitor concentrate infusion has been effective in the management of acute angio-oedema; danazol, an androgen, has been effective in the long-term prophylaxis of angio-oedema. Danazol is unsuitable for children and pregnant women because of its androgenic effects (e.g. hirsutism).
- Life-threatening anaphylaxis requires urgent intervention (Table 16.4) followed by a course of oral steroids and an anti-histamine. Individuals with a history of anaphylaxis should be advised to wear a MedicAlert® bracelet and carry an EpiPen® (containing 1:1000 adrenaline 300μg 0.3mL [adult dose]). The patient and a family member should be taught how to administer intramuscular adrenaline via an EpiPen® in the event of anaphylaxis.

Necrotising fasciitis

Necrotising fasciitis (also called 'flesh-eating disease') is an uncommon, potentially life-threatening soft tissue infection. The most common causative organism is Group A Streptococcus. It is characterised by painful, rapidly progressive skin swelling, colour changes from red to purple–grey and subsequent necrosis of subcutaneous tissue and fascia. Patients become toxic with fever, tachycardia and septic shock. Old age, diabetes, non-healing ulcers, penetrating trauma and surgery predispose to necrotising fasciitis.

Management
- Investigations include full blood count, renal function, C-reactive protein and wound swabs for bacterial culture.
- Broad-spectrum intravenous antibiotics and surgical debridement of necrotic tissue is the mainstay of treatment.
- Fluid and electrolyte replacement, nutritional support and analgesia.

> **Key points**
> - Dermatological emergencies can be potentially life-threatening.
> - Most common causes are underlying skin diseases or drugs.
> - Principles of the management of most dermatological emergencies include identifying and treating or withdrawing the underlying cause, supportive care in a high-dependency environment and prevention of complications.
> - Individuals with a history of angio-oedema and anaphylaxis should wear a MedicAlert® bracelet and carry an EpiPen®.

> ► **Warning**
>
> In view of the large surface area of skin loss and consequent life-threatening complications, patients with TEN are best managed in a high-dependency setting or burns unit.

Table 17.1 Possible causes of skin blistering

- **Inherited**: e.g. epidermolysis bullosa (see Chapter 46), bullous ichthyosiform erythroderma (see Chapter 46), bullous cutaneous porphyrias (see Chapter 40)
- **Acquired**:
  - drug-induced: e.g. fixed drug eruption, Stevens-Johnson syndrome toxic epidermal necrolysis (see Chapter 16)
  - infections: e.g. bullous impetigo, staphylococcal scalded skin syndrome (see Chapter 27)
  - autoimmune: e.g. linear IgA disease (see Chapter 27), bullous pemphigoid, pemphigus, dermatitis herpetiformis
  - other: insect bites, severe sunburn, phytophotodermatitis

Fig. 17.1 Schematic diagram of the skin basement membrane

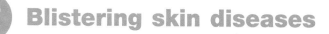

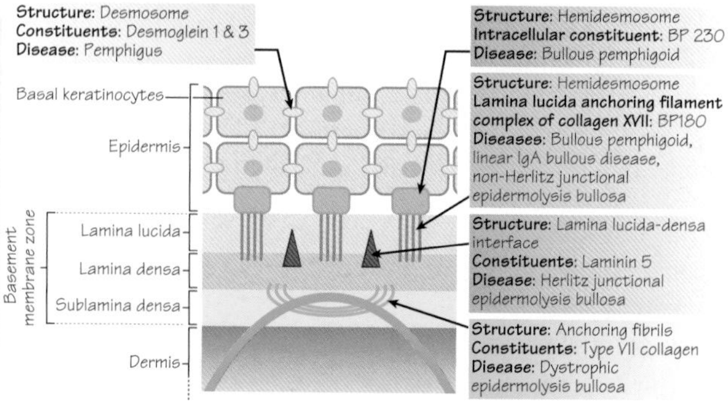

Structure: Desmosome
Constituents: Desmoglein 1 & 3
Disease: Pemphigus

Structure: Hemidesmosome
Intracellular constituent: BP 230
Disease: Bullous pemphigoid

Structure: Hemidesmosome
Lamina lucida anchoring filament complex of collagen XVII: BP180
Diseases: Bullous pemphigoid, linear IgA bullous disease, non-Herlitz junctional epidermolysis bullosa

Structure: Lamina lucida-densa interface
Constituents: Laminin 5
Disease: Herlitz junctional epidermolysis bullosa

Structure: Anchoring fibrils
Constituents: Type VII collagen
Disease: Dystrophic epidermolysis bullosa

Basal keratinocytes
Epidermis
Basement membrane zone
Lamina lucida
Lamina densa
Sublamina densa
Dermis

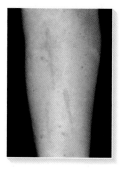

Fig. 17.2
Phytophoto-dermatitis – note the linear urticated lesions and nearby blisters

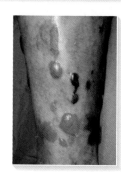

Fig. 17.3
Bullous pemphigoid – note the tense blisters, some of which are haemorrhagic, that burst to leave superficial erosions on the skin

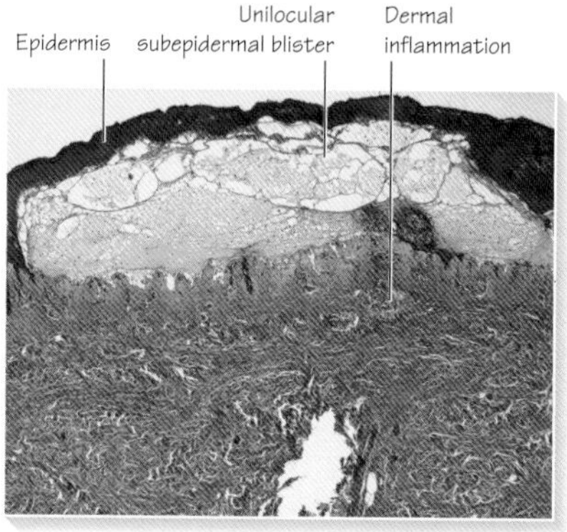

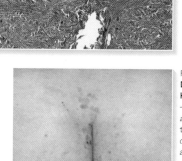

Epidermis Unilocular subepidermal blister Dermal inflammation

Fig. 17.4
Histology of bullous pemphigoid – note the subepidermal blister on this H&E stain x4

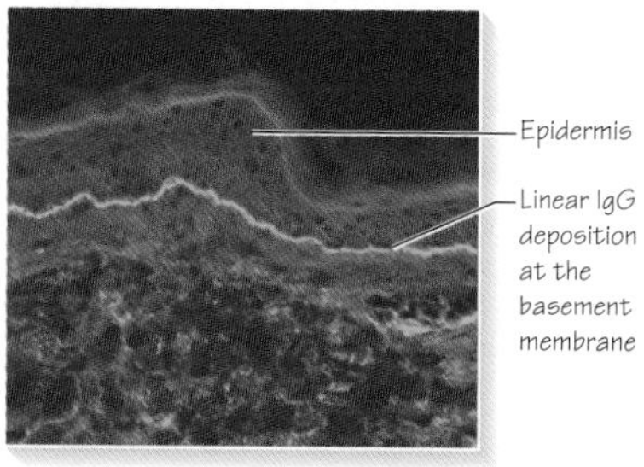

Fig. 17.5
Direct immunofluorescence of bullous pemphigoid – note the linear deposition of IgG at the basement membrane

Epidermis

Linear IgG deposition at the basement membrane

Fig. 17.6a/b
Pemphigus vulgaris – blisters are fragile and therefore often erosions and crusting are seen rather than blisters

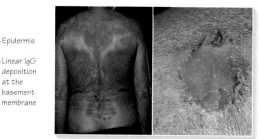

Fig. 17.7
Dermatitis herpetiformis – itchy vesicles and small blisters typically develop on the buttocks and extensor aspects of the limbs

Table 17.2 Differentiating features between bullous skin diseases

Disease	Clinical features	Aetiology	Histology	Direct immunofluorescence
Bullous pemphigoid	Tense blisters on an urticated base	IgG autoantibodies to basement membrane antigen BP180 or BP230	Subepidermal blisters (Fig 17.4)	Linear IgG at the basement membrane
Pemphigus	Flaccid blisters, skin erosions and crusting +/– mucosal involvement	Autoantibodies to epidermal cell surface proteins desmoglein 1 and 3	Intraepidermal acantholysis +/– blisters	Cell surface bound IgG, net-like pattern in epidermis
Dermatitis herpetiformis	Itchy small blisters & vesicles	IgA autoantibodies to gluten tissue transaminase in the gut and epidermis	Subepidermal blisters	Granular IgA in dermal papillary tips

Table 17.3 Differentiating features between the types of pemphigus

Type of pemphigus	Skin involvement	Mucosal surface involvement	Circulating auto-antibodies to	Histology
Pemphigus vulgaris	Fragile blisters & erosions	Always involved	Desmoglein 1 & 3	Suprabasal acantholysis
Pemphigus foliaceus	Superficial scaly erosions	Spared	Desmoglein 1	Subcorneal acantholysis
Paraneoplastic pemphigus	Skin erosions	Severe	Desmoglein 1 & 3, desmoplakin	Suprabasal acantholysis

Dermatology at a Glance, First Edition. Mahbub M.U. Chowdhury, Ruwani P. Katugampola, and Andrew Y. Finlay.

The skin may blister as a result of different causes (Table 17.1). Disruption of the complex skin basement membrane (BM) at different levels leads to the different blistering skin diseases (Figure 17.1).

The most common causes of blistering are insect bites and severe sunburn. Phytophotodermatitis is an uncommon blistering rash caused by a phototoxic reaction following sunlight exposure after contact with plants containing photosensitising chemicals such as psoralen (e.g. giant hogweed, celery, parsnip and rue). Painful and/or itchy urticated plaques or blisters appear within 24 hours of contact in a streaky pattern at the sites of plant contact (Figure 17.2). Management is with potent topical corticosteroids and antihistamines and avoiding future contact with offending plants.

Autoimmune bullous skin diseases

Autoantibodies against epidermis or BM components lead to activation of an inflammatory cascade with cleavage of the skin at different levels and blistering (Figure 17.1). Diagnosis is made clinically and confirmed by histology (Table 17.2).

Investigations include serum antibodies to target antigen, biopsy lesional skin for haematoxylin and eosinophil staining (differentiates level of skin cleavage causing the blister), peri-lesional skin for direct immunofluorescence (IMF) and serum for indirect IMF.

Immunofluorescence

IMF helps to differentiate between types of bullous diseases.

Direct IMF A fluorescein-labelled antibody against the suspect disease-causing antibody and/or complement is added to the peri-lesional skin biopsy from the patient. When examined under UV light it demonstrates the deposition pattern of autoantibodies and complement in the skin characteristic of the different bullous skin diseases (Table 17.2).

Indirect IMF The patient's serum containing the disease-causing antibodies are added to an animal tissue (e.g. monkey oesophagus), incubated and highlighted under UV light using fluorescein-labelled anti-human antibody.

Bullous pemphigoid

Bullous pemphigoid is an autoimmune bullous disease which is more common in elderly people.

Symptoms and signs Intense pruritus may precede the onset of tense (as the blister wall is the complete epidermis) blisters on an erythematous background which may be localised or widespread (Figure 17.3). Blisters may also occur on mucosal surfaces (e.g. oral mucosa). The blisters later burst to leave superficial erosions that heal without scarring.

Aetiology Immunoglobulin G (IgG) autoantibodies to BM antigens BP180 (type XVII collagen) or BP230 result in cleavage of the skin at the dermo-epidermal junction leading to subepidermal blisters (Figures 17.4 and 17.5).

Investigations See above and Table 17.2.

Treatment Localised disease is treated with topical super-potent corticosteroids (e.g. 0.05% clobetasol propionate). Widespread disease requires a reducing course of oral prednisolone starting at about 30–40 mg/day combined with an oral immunosuppressant (e.g. azathioprine, mycophenolate mofetil) or tetracycline in combination with nicotinamide.

Pemphigus

Pemphigus comprises a group of rare, potentially life-threatening, autoimmune bullous skin diseases which usually affect middle-aged individuals.

Aetiology IgG autoantibodies to epidermal cell surface proteins desmoglein 1 and 3 lead to loss of cell–cell adhesion (acantholysis) at different levels of the epidermis causing flaccid blisters or scaly erosions of the skin (Figures 17.6a,b) and/or mucous membranes. Blisters are fragile as the blister wall is the thin upper part of the epidermis.

Signs and symptoms The three main types of pemphigus are summarised in Table 17.3. Paraneoplastic pemphigus occurs in association with an underlying lympho-proliferative disease (e.g. non-Hodgkin's lymphoma, Castleman's disease, thymoma).

Investigations See above and Table 17.2. Paraneoplastic pemphigus should prompt investigation for an underlying malignancy (e.g. full blood count, blood film, chest X-ray, further radiological studies such as chest CT scan).

Treatment Systemic therapy with high-dose weaning course of oral steroids (e.g. 60 mg/day prednisolone) in combination with an immunosuppressant (e.g. azathioprine, mycophenolate mofetil). Other treatments include intravenous immunoglobulin, cyclophosphamide and rituximab.

Dermatitis herpetiformis

This is an autoimmune bullous skin disease usually affecting young and middle-aged individuals due to IgA autoantibodies (also called IgA anti-endomysial antibodies) to gluten tissue trans-glutaminase in the gut and epidermis. The male:female ratio is 2:1.

Signs and symptoms Itchy vesicles or small blisters, typically on the extensor aspects of limbs and buttocks. Because of the intense itch, excoriations may be the only sign seen (Figure 17.7). Approximately 75% of patients may also give a history of gluten-sensitive enteropathy (coeliac disease).

Investigations See above and Table 17.2. Direct IMF in dermatitis herpetiformis shows granular IgA deposition in dermal papillary tips in contrast to linear IgA disease (see Chapter 27) where linear IgA deposition is seen along the epidermal BM.

Treatment Oral dapsone and gluten-free diet. Dapsone rapidly relieves itch. Blood glucose-6-phosphate dehydrogenase level needs to be checked as its deficiency increases the risk of haemolysis due to dapsone. Patients on dapsone require monitoring of full blood count and reticulocyte count (risk of haemolytic anaemia) and liver function (risk of hepatotoxicity).

> ### Key points
> - Intense pruritus may precede the onset of blisters in bullous pemphigoid and dermatitis herpetiformis.
> - IMF is essential to diagnose autoimmune bullous diseases.
> - Mucosal surfaces may be affected in blistering skin diseases.

> ### ► Warning
> Patients on long-term high-dose oral steroids need osteoporosis prophylaxis and monitoring for steroid-induced hypertension and diabetes (glycosuria and raised serum glucose).

Table 18.1
Other skin bacterial infections

- Staphylococcal Scalded Skin Syndrome (see Chapter 27)
- Staphylococcal infection in atopic dermatitis (see Chapter 13)
- Syphilis (see Chapter 24)
- Leishmaniasis (see Chapter 22)

Table 18.2
Diseases involving the skin caused by spirochaetes

- Syphilis
- Lyme disease
- Yaws

Fig. 18.1 **Cellulitis: spreading erythema**

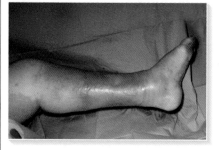

▶ **Warning**

Differential diagnosis of a hot red leg includes cellulitis, deep venous thrombosis and lipodermatosclerosis.

Fig. 18.2 **Erysipelas of face**

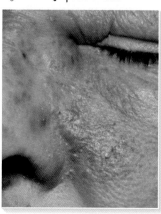

Fig. 18.3 **Impetigo**

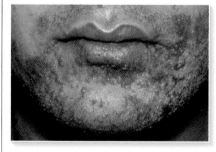

Fig. 18.4 **Folliculitis**

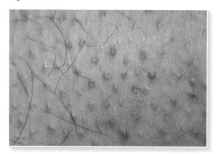

Fig. 18.5 **Healing furuncle (boil)**

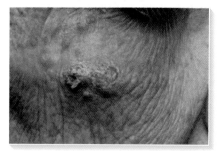

Fig. 18.6 **Intertrigo: inflammation in skin folds**

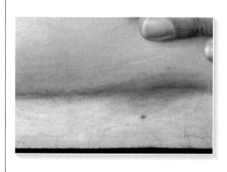

Fig. 18.7 **Pitted keratolysis: 'moth-eaten' appearance**

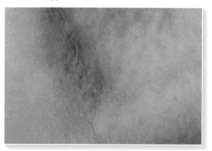

Fig. 18.8 **Fish tank granuloma between fingers with proximal spread**

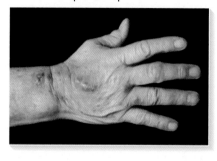

Skin is covered by billions of 'normal' commensal bacteria that prevent pathogenic organisms becoming established. But bacterial skin infections are highly prevalent, and without antibiotics may be fatal. It is important to recognise and treat them early.

Avoidance of infection confers survival advantage: fear of skin disease 'Is it catching, doctor?' is therefore 'sensible'.

Common bacteria causing infection include *Staphylococcus aureus, Streptococcus pyogenes, Corynebacterium minutissimum, Mycobacterium tuberculosis, Mycobacterium marinum* and *Spirochaetes*.

Cellulitis and erysipelas

- Redness, swelling, heat, tenderness, pyrexia.
- Take swabs for culture from fluid or cracked areas.
- Treatment: 500 mg flucloxacillin four times daily.
- Risks: recurrence, lymphoedema.

Cellulitis (Figure 18.1) *Streptococcus* group A or *Staphylococcus aureus* infection of subcutaneous tissue, typically of lower leg. Diffuse edge.

Erysipelas (Figure 18.2) *Streptococcus* group A infection of the dermis. Typically well-defined with red raised edge, on the face, with initial infection around nose or ears.

Impetigo (Figure 18.3)

Superficial infection of epidermis, redness and crusting usually of face in children. Easily infects other children. Non-bullous impetigo is usually caused by *Staphylococcus aureus* (*aureus* means 'gold' – the colour of the culture) or by *Streptococcus pyogenes*. *Staphyloccocus aureus* causes bullous impetigo with blistering.

Treatment: topical mupirocin, systemic flucloxacillin or erythromycin. If undiagnosed impetigo is treated wrongly with topical steroids, it initially improves but then gets worse.

Folliculitis (Figure 18.4)

Very common inflammation around hair follicles resulting in small itchy red pustules on scalp or body. Pustules may be sterile or may grow coagulase-negative *Staphylococci* or *Staphylococcus aureus*. Predisposing factors include topical irritants and occlusion. Check local and nasal swabs.

Treatment: may settle by itself, but can be persistent and difficult to cure. If severe and *Staphylococci* isolated, topical mupirocin or systemic flucloxacillin. If nasal swabs positive, treat nostrils with mupirocin to reduce nasal carriage.

Boil (furuncle) (Figure 18.5)

Hair follicle infection from *Staphylococcus aureus* and nasal carriage. Like a volcano, if the 'head' is broken pus gushes out.

Treatment: flucloxacillin. If recurrent, check for diabetes, HIV or Panton–Valentine leukocidin (PVL) toxin strain of *Staphylococcus*.

Erythrasma

Bacterial infection caused by *Corynebacterium minutissimum* (*minutissimum* means 'very small'). Diffuse persisting symptomless rash in toe webs, groin or axillae, that under Wood's light (UVA 365 nm) fluoresces 'coral red'. Differential diagnosis fungal infection.

Treatment: very sensitive to a wide range of topical antibiotics and also sensitive to azoles (e.g. clotrimazole).

Intertrigo (Figure 18.6)

Inflammation of the skin in the body folds (e.g. beneath breasts). Stratum corneum always touching so folds of the skin are moist, creating a warm environment liked by bacteria and fungi. A 'soup' of organisms gives a red sore itchy smelly oozing rash.

Treatment: keep body folds apart and dry with dressings. Apply topical antibiotic anti-fungal low potency steroid mixtures.

Pitted keratolysis (Figure 18.7)

'Moth-eaten' appearance of soles caused by *Corynebacterium* and other bacteria. Smelly sore superficial erosions, associated with excessive sweating (hyperhidrosis).

Treatment: fucidin ointment and treat the hyperhidrosis.

Trichomycosis axillaris

Thickening and nodules of hair in axillae, caused by gram-positive *Corynebacteria*. Not fungal, despite its fungus-sounding name. Common in males, but usually symptom free.

Treatment: antiperspirant anhydrous aluminium chloride, shave hair.

Tuberculosis

Direct infection If there is high host immunity: lupus vulgaris ('common wolf'), a single red–brown plaque on head or neck, or warty tuberculosis, a thick warty plaque at area of trauma. If there is poor host immunity: scrofuloderma, an ulcerating nodule over a lymph gland.

Secondary effects Erythema nodosum or erythema induratum (a 'tuberculid'), nodules that may ulcerate over the back of the lower legs in women.

Suspected tuberculosis must be fully investigated locally with skin biopsy for culture and systemically with chest X-ray. In the UK, TB is a notifiable disease. Seek advice from other specialists about investigation and treatment.

Fish-tank granuloma (Figure 18.8)

Tropical fish owners scratch hands on rocks when cleaning their fish tanks. A persistant purple plaque develops after 3 weeks, because of an 'atypical' *Mycobacterium marinum* infection.

Treatment: biopsy and culture, then doxycycline or clarithromycin.

Lyme disease

Borrelia burgdorferi infection via tick bites, often from deer, while walking in woodland. Named after Lyme, Connecticut. Erythema chronicum migrans, an enlarging red circle, starts a week after the bite and may persist for months. Systemic features: arthritis 50%, neurological 20%, cardiac 10%. Diagnosis by antibody response.

Treatment: 100 mg doxycycline three times daily for 2–3 weeks. Oral treatment is essential to prevent systemic problems.

Key points

- Correct diagnosis of infections is essential.
- Topical steroids make infection worse.
- If signs of cellulitis or erysipelas, systemic antibiotics are essential.

19 Viral infections

Fig. 19.1a/b **Warts on hands/fingers**

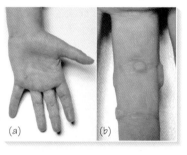

(a) (b)

Fig. 19.1c/d **Plantar warts**

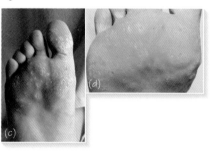

(c) (d)

Fig. 19.1e **Viral wart with bleeding points** (capillaries)

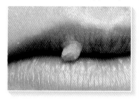

Fig. 19.1f **Wart on upper lip**

Fig. 19.2a/b **Periungual viral wart**

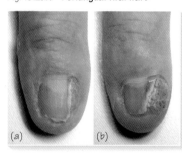

(a) (b)

Fig. 19.3a/b **Herpes simplex virus (HSV)** keratitis/ulcers seen with slit lamp

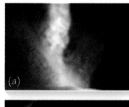

(a)

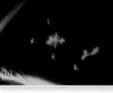

(b)

Fig. 19.4a/b **Neonatal eczema herpeticum on face**

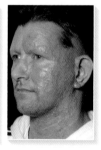

(a) (b)

Fig. 19.4c **HSV infection on adult face**

Fig. 19.5a **HSV around lips**

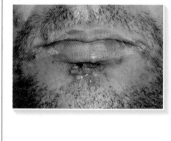

Fig. 19.5b **HSV on hand**

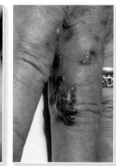

Fig. 19.5c **HSV fingers** – note haemorrhagic areas

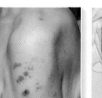

Fig. 19.6a **Herpes zoster infection on arm**

Fig. 19.6b **Herpes zoster on leg**

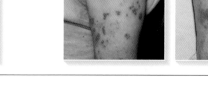

Viral infections are extremely common and can affect a wide range of ages including young children. They vary in seriousness and how aggressive treatment needs to be depends on the clinical presentation and symptoms. The common viral infections presenting to GPs and dermatologists are discussed here.

Viral warts

Common viral warts are caused by the human papilloma virus types 1, 2 and 4 and can present on the fingers, hands and feet (Figure 19.1). Plane (flat) warts may also occur on the dorsum of the hands and face. Typically, warts have dark pinpoint areas which are thrombosed capillaries more obvious when the wart is pared down (Figure 19.1e). This sign is essential to differentiate a wart from an area of callus that could be mistakenly treated as a wart.

Warts are usually asymptomatic and treatment is not essential, particularly in children. In children, the pain of liquid nitrogen cryotherapy is usually not tolerated. Warts around the nail folds (Figure 19.2) or plantar warts can be treated with salicyclic acid-based preparations which cannot be used on the face.

In adults presenting with multiple warts, immunosuppression should be considered including HIV infection. Patients on long-term immunosuppressives such as azathioprine and ciclosporin can also be affected. Adults are likely to tolerate more aggressive treatment such as cryotherapy or curettage.

Genital warts are treated usually in the genito-urinary department with topical imiquimod or podophyllotoxin.

Hyperkeratotic warts are ideally pared down to remove the thickening prior to any treatments.

Herpes infections

Herpes simplex

Herpes simplex (cold sore) presents as painful grouped vesicles and erosions caused by human herpes virus 1 or 2. In children, herpes simplex may be asymptomatic or cause fever and regional lymphadenopathy. In neonates, there may be gingivitis, keratoconjunctivitis or herpes labialis. This will need management with other specialists, particularly for the eyes (Figure 19.3) and genital areas. Differential diagnoses include herpes zoster, impetigo and other dermatoses.

Eczema herpeticum is a dermatological emergency. It is a widespread infection with herpes simplex in a patient with previous atopic eczema and should always be excluded in an acute severe exacerbation of stable eczema. Patients present with multiple crusted and vesicular lesions, often on the face (Figure 19.4). This can frequently be confused with a bacterial infection or a flare-up of the eczema itself.

In adults, herpes simplex can affect the peri-oral area and also the fingers (Figure 19.5). It can also provoke erythema multiforme. If herpes simplex is recurrent, prophylaxis with continuous anti-viral treatments such as oral aciclovir for 3–6 months may be required, especially with presentations such as erythema multiforme.

Herpes zoster

Herpes zoster (shingles) is an acute vesicular eruption, usually within a single dermatome, resulting from reactivation of vari-cella zoster virus from a previous infection with chickenpox (Figure 19.6). The rash heals spontaneously within 2–3 weeks; however, it may leave scarring. Herpes zoster infection should be considered if there is a painful blistering eruption occurring in one or several dermatomes. You can 'catch' chickenpox from herpes zoster if you have not previously had chickenpox.

Herpes zoster affecting the eye needs to be treated urgently to prevent problems such as keratitis and, if left untreated, blindness.

Investigations

Diagnosis of herpes simplex and herpes zoster is usually obvious clinically but in atypical cases investigations such as herpes serology are necessary.

To diagnose atypical presentations of viral infections, electron microscopy of blister fluid, viral culture from swab of a lesion (Table 19.2) and skin biopsy are essential. For herpes zoster, specific investigations include viral culture, serology, electron microscopy, Tzanck smear (Table 19.3) and checking HIV status if appropriate.

Treatment

For herpes simplex, 200 mg oral aciclovir five times per day for 5 days is used. Herpes zoster is treated with intravenous or oral aciclovir or valciclovir to prevent progression and reduce risk of post-herpetic neuralgia which can be chronic and extremely painful and debilitating. Oral aciclovir is poorly absorbed (only 20%) and hence high doses are needed for herpes zoster, 200 mg five times daily for at least 7 days. Failure to respond to aciclovir may be due to poor absorption or rapid clearance following ingestion or possibly aciclovir resistance. Valciclovir and famciclovir are alternatives with improved bioavailability. Side effects include headache, nausea, diarrhoea, renal, hepatic and neurological dysfunction.

All antiviral agents need to be used within 24–48 hours of eruptions commencing, in either herpes simplex or herpes zoster. Post-herpetic neuralgia treatments such as analgesics and narcotics may not be effective (Table 19.1).

Molluscum contagiosum

See Chapter 27.

Key points

- Herpes simplex and herpes zoster need to be treated within 1–2 days of vesicular lesions.
- Check HIV status in all patients with atypical herpes or viral infections.
- If aciclovir is ineffective remember resistance may occur.

▶ **Warning**

Beware eczema herpeticum in any acute severe flare-up of eczema presenting with vesicles, especially on the face.

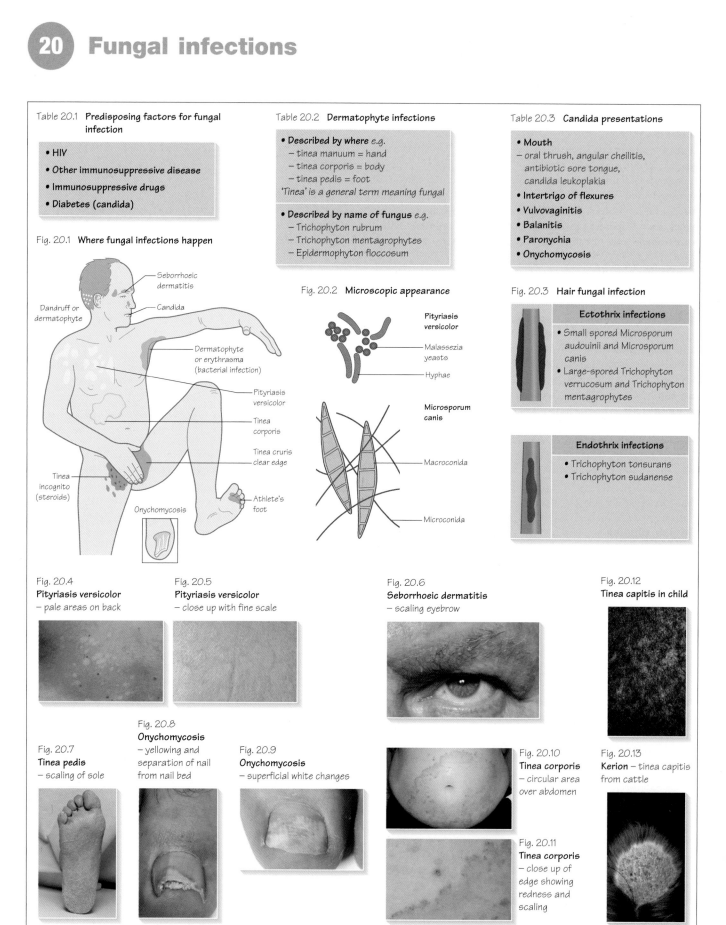

Table 20.1 **Predisposing factors for fungal infection**

- HIV
- Other immunosuppressive disease
- Immunosuppressive drugs
- Diabetes (candida)

Fig. 20.1 **Where fungal infections happen**

Seborrhoeic dermatitis

Dandruff or dermatophyte

Candida

Dermatophyte or erythrasma (bacterial infection)

Pityriasis versicolor

Tinea corporis

Tinea cruris clear edge

Tinea incognito (steroids)

Onychomycosis

Athlete's foot

Table 20.2 **Dermatophyte infections**

- **Described by where** *e.g.*
  - tinea manuum = hand
  - tinea corporis = body
  - tinea pedis = foot
  'Tinea' is a general term meaning fungal

- **Described by name of fungus** *e.g.*
  - Trichophyton rubrum
  - Trichophyton mentagrophytes
  - Epidermophyton floccosum

Fig. 20.2 **Microscopic appearance**

Pityriasis versicolor

Malassezia yeasts

Hyphae

Microsporum canis

Macroconida

Microconida

Table 20.3 **Candida presentations**

- Mouth
  - oral thrush, angular cheilitis, antibiotic sore tongue, candida leukoplakia
- Intertrigo of flexures
- Vulvovaginitis
- Balanitis
- Paronychia
- Onychomycosis

Fig. 20.3 **Hair fungal infection**

Ectothrix infections

- Small spored Microsporum audouinii and Microsporum canis
- Large-spored Trichophyton verrucosum and Trichophyton mentagrophytes

Endothrix infections

- Trichophyton tonsurans
- Trichophyton sudanense

Fig. 20.4 **Pityriasis versicolor** – pale areas on back

Fig. 20.5 **Pityriasis versicolor** – close up with fine scale

Fig. 20.6 **Seborrhoeic dermatitis** – scaling eyebrow

Fig. 20.12 **Tinea capitis in child**

Fig. 20.7 **Tinea pedis** – scaling of sole

Fig. 20.8 **Onychomycosis** – yellowing and separation of nail from nail bed

Fig. 20.9 **Onychomycosis** – superficial white changes

Fig. 20.10 **Tinea corporis** – circular area over abdomen

Fig. 20.11 **Tinea corporis** – close up of edge showing redness and scaling

Fig. 20.13 **Kerion** – tinea capitis from cattle

Dermatology at a Glance, First Edition. Mahbub M.U. Chowdhury, Ruwani P. Katugampola, and Andrew Y. Finlay.

There are two main types of fungi. Moulds (e.g. dermatophytes) have long hyphae and grow from the tip. Yeasts (e.g. *Malassezia* and *Candida*) are single-celled organisms, shaped like rugby balls or footballs, that bud to produce new cells (Figure 20.2).

Pityriasis versicolor (Figures 20.4 and 20.5)

Multiple patches coalesce over upper back, shoulders and chest in young adults, with light scaling, seen if gently scraped with spatula. 'Pityriasis' indicates fine scale, 'versicolor' means variable colour change: some areas become lighter, others darker. Caused by overgrowth of normal skin commensal lipophilic yeasts *Malassezia globosa*, *Malassezia sympodialis* and *Malassezia furfur*.

Treatment: ketoconazole shampoo applied three times or 2.5% selenium sulphide (Selsun® shampoo) applied on alternate nights for a week. Oral 200 mg/day itraconazole for 5 days if widespread.

Malassezia folliculitis

Itchy papules and pustules on the back and upper body are seen in young adults. The differential diagnosis acne is not itchy.

Treatment: as for pityriasis versicolor.

Seborrhoeic dermatitis, dandruff

Superficial scaling in the sternal area, eyebrows (Figure 20.6), ears, nasolabial folds and diffusely throughout scalp is seen. Adult seborrhoeic dermatitis is caused by *Malassezia* species.

Treatment: as for pityriasis versicolor.

Dermatophyte infections

Tinea pedis ('athlete's foot') (Figure 20.7)

The most common fungal infection, spread by walking in communal changing rooms. Macerated skin between the fourth and fifth toes is seen; it may involve other toe webs, the sole or dorsum of the foot. Vesicles may coalesce, forming bullae because of thick stratum corneum. Usually caused by *Trichophyton rubrum*.

Onychomycosis or tinea unguium (nails) (Figs. 20.8, 20.9)

Yellow–brown crumbly thickened nails are seen, infected from tinea pedis. The most common organisms are *Trichophyton rubrum*, *Trichophyton mentagrophytes* or *Epidermophyton floccosum*. If nail clippings show hyphae on microscopy or grow dermatophytes, treat with 250 mg/day terbinafine for 12 weeks.

Tinea cruris (groin)

This has superficial itchy scaling with a well-defined edge. There may be other co-existing infections, such as *Candida* or erythrasma. Topical azoles are also effective against *Candida* so consider using if *Candida* is also suspected.

Tinea corporis (body) (Figures 20.10 and 20.11)

Circular lesions are seen, hence 'ringworm' (no worm but remember the ring), which may coalesce and show central clearing. Scrape slightly scaly edge for microscopy and culture.

Tinea capitis (scalp, also including hair) (Figures 20.3, 20.12)

The fungus may be on the outside of the hair (ectothrix). It may invade the full shaft thickness (endothrix) making the shaft much weaker and so hairs break easily, giving patchy baldness with black dots, the broken ends.

The epidemiology constantly changes. *Trichophyton tonsurans* is now common in UK and USA urban areas, and *Microsporum canis* is common in some European countries.

Kerion (Figure 20.13)

An area of severe inflammation, usually on the scalp, caused by a zoophilic dermatophyte (i.e. whose host is normally an animal). As the organism has not evolved on human skin, there is a severe reaction (e.g. *Trichophyton verrucosum* from cattle).

Treatment: 10 mg/kg griseofulvin daily for 6 weeks.

Favus

Favus is a distinctive type of tinea capitis with yellow cup-shaped crusts (scutula), caused by *Trichophyton schoenleinii*. Endemic in South Africa and Ethiopia, it may cause scarring alopecia.

Investigations for fungal infections

• *Skin:* scrape edge of active lesions into folded paper or cardboard. Dermatophytes and yeasts may remain alive for weeks.
• *Hair:* pull out hairs with forceps and culture. Or brush a disposable toothbrush through the affected area 10 times, then press the brush into culture medium in a Petri dish.
• *Nail:* clip nail, including soft matter beneath protruding edge.
• *Wood's light:* UVA (365 nm) shows extent of pityriasis versicolor. Causes fluorescence of hair in some dermatophyte infections (e.g. *Microsporum canis*). Useful for screening in a school outbreak. Skin dermatophyte infection does not fluoresce.

Dermatophyte infection treatment

Terbinafine 1% cream is fungicidal so even one application can cure. If applied daily for 5 days, less areas will be missed. Terbinafine inhibits squalene epoxidase in fungal cells, so squalene levels build up and they become deficient in ergosterol, essential for fungal (but not human) cell membranes. Other topical treatments for dermatophyte infections include the imidazoles (e.g. ketoconazole, miconazole, clotrimazole) and cheaper treatment such as benzoic acid (Whitfield's) ointment.

Candida infection

Candida albicans is the most common *Candida* species and is a normal commensal in the mouth and gut. Albicans means 'white': both the cultured yeast and the appearance of thrush look white. Superficial *Candida* infections affect the skin (sometimes with pustules) and nail folds (*Candida paronychia*). Infection of the mouth ('oral thrush') may be the presenting sign of HIV. Diabetes may predispose to skin *Candida* infections. Treatment is with topical imidazoles or oral fluconazole or itraconazole.

> **Key points**
> • The key sign of fungal infections is superficial scaling.
> • Toe webs are the main site for dermatophyte infections. Check them if fungal infection elsewhere suspected.

> ▶ **Warning**
>
> • Both tinea and Trichophyton are abbreviated to 'T'.
> • Topical steroids settle itch so seem to be helpful, but fungus grows better, resulting in tinea incognito ('in disguise'). Don't use steroids in fungal infections.

Fig. 21.1
Crusted scabies of the foot

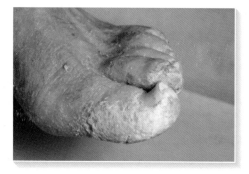

Scabies

Scabies is caused by the mite *Sarcoptes scabiei*. Spread is by direct person-to-person contact. The adult female mite burrows into the stratum corneum where she lays her eggs. The eggs hatch after a few days in the stratum corneum where the larvae mature into adult mites within two weeks and the female mites lay their eggs to continue the cycle.

The symptoms and signs occur about 4 weeks after infestation, because of a hypersensitivity reaction to the mites: intensely itchy skin with irregular slightly scaly burrows (seen between the finger webs, wrists, ankles, medial and lateral borders of feet) and papules (seen on the penis). In infants, the face is often affected with red itchy papules and hands and feet with vesicles. A secondary eczematous rash is often seen a few weeks after treatment.

Crusted scabies (previously called Norwegian scabies) is severe infestation with scabies resulting in hyperkeratosis of the skin including the subungual skin (Figure 21.1). This is seen in cases of untreated scabies (e.g. elderly individuals with dementia) or those with immune deficiency (e.g. immunosuppression following organ transplantation or in HIV infection).

Diagnosis is based on the clinical features described above. With a magnifying glass, the mite may be visible as a white dot at the end of the burrow. Close contacts should also be examined for scabies.

Management includes simultaneous treatment of the index case as well as their close contacts (e.g. partner and family members) with topical insecticides, either 5% permethrin cream or 0.5% malathion liquid (safer option in pregnant women and children), two applications 1 week apart. The treatment is applied to the whole body (neck to toes in adults, treat face and scalp as well in infants) and left on for 24 hours. Schools or other institutions (e.g. care homes) attended by the infested individual should be informed as a matter of priority to identify and prevent further spread of the infestation.

Crusted scabies is treated with oral ivermectin. Clothing and bed linen of the index case and their close contacts should be washed at high temperature (50°C).

Head lice (pediculosis capitis)

Head lice are caused by the arthropod *Pediculus humanus capitis*. It is the most common parasitic infestation in school children. The school or nursery attended by the infested child should be informed as a matter of priority, to identify and prevent further spread of the infestation. Infestation is confined to the scalp and is spread by direct head-to-head contact. It can also spread via clothes, hair brushes and bed clothing.

The louse has three pairs of clawed legs adapted to grasping the hair shaft. The female lice lay their eggs (nits), which are firmly attached to the host's hair. The eggs hatch after about 7–10 days and the cycle continues. The louse feeds on its host's blood while injecting its saliva into the host.

Head lice infestation may be asymptomatic. However, some experience intense itching associated with excoriations, eczematous rash and impetiginisation of the scalp and cervical lymphadenopathy about 1 month after the initial infestation. This is due to hypersensitivity to the saliva injected by the louse.

Severe untreated head lice infestation may present with marked hyperkeratosis of the scalp with thick scales adherent to the hair shafts (pityriasis amiantacea). The differential diagnoses include severe scalp psoriasis and fungal scalp infection (tinea capitis).

The diagnosis of head lice is made clinically, by examination of the scalp aided by a magnifying glass to identify nits attached to the hair shafts, often proximally, and crawling lice. The scalp of close contacts should also be examined for head lice.

Simultaneous treatment of the index case and their close contacts (e.g. family members) is needed. Treatment includes wet combing with topical insecticides to kill the lice and nits. Wet combing involves the mechanical removal of lice and nits. The wet hair is combed for about 15–30 minutes with a fine toothed comb daily for 2 weeks until no further lice are seen.

Topical therapy includes 0.5% malathion lotion (safer in pregnant women and children) which is applied to the hair, washed off after 12 hours and repeated 1 week later. An alternative is 1% permethrin cream, applied to damp towel-dried hair and rinsed off after 10 minutes and repeated 1 week later. Clothing and bed linen of the index case and their close contacts should be washed at high temperature (50°C). Hair combs and brushes of these individuals and toys should be disinfected.

Body lice

Body lice are caused by the arthropod *Pediculus humanus corporis* and may be seen in self-neglected individuals. Spread is by direct person-to-person contact. Management as for scabies.

Key points

Topical malathion is the preferred treatment for scabies or head lice in pregnant women and children.

▶ Warning

Scabies and head lice spread from person to person. Treat close contacts at the same time as the patient.

Fig. 22.1 **Cutaneous larva migrans** – note the characteristic extending serpiginous track

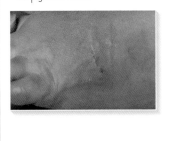

Fig. 22.2 **Cutaneous leishmaniasis**

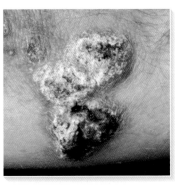

Fig. 22.3 **Leprosy**
(a) note erythematous plaque on bridge of nose and thickened right supratrochlear nerve
(b) note anaesthetic hypopigmented macular patch over right deltoid region

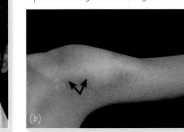

Cutaneous larva migrans

Caused by hookworm larvae in soil contaminated by animal faeces. The larvae penetrate and migrate into the human skin, especially via sites in contact with contaminated soil (e.g. feet, buttocks). Patients present with an extremely itchy, erythematous, serpiginous track that extends over days due to larval movement (Figure 22.1). The track consists of a combination of papules, vesicles or blisters. Diagnosis is made clinically. The condition is self-limiting as larvae die within 6–8 weeks of penetrating the skin. Treatment of limited disease is with topical 10% thiabendazole cream for 1–2 weeks; if widespread disease, oral albendazole or ivermectin.

Leishmaniasis

Caused by different species of the protozoan parasite, *Leishmania*. It is transmitted by infected female sandflies who bite human hosts and pass the protozoans into their bloodstream. Incubation period ranges from weeks to a year. There are three main types:
1 **Cutaneous** is the most common form. Patients present with one or more painless ulcers (termed tropical ulcers; Figure 22.2) on exposed skin, often the face or limb, which heals over months with scarring. Regional lymphadenopathy may be present.
2 **Mucocutaneous** form, occurs months or years after healing of a cutaneous leishmaniasis lesion. May lead to partial or complete destruction of mucous membranes (e.g. nasopharynx).
3 **Visceral form (kala azar)** is the most severe, due to visceral organ involvement. Patients present with fever, weight loss, hepatosplenomegaly and anaemia. Mortality in untreated cases is >90%. Also occurs as opportunistic infection associated with HIV infection.

About 90% of visceral leishmaniasis occurs in the Indian subcontinent, Sudan, Ethiopia and Brazil; 90% of cutaneous leishmaniasis is in Afghanistan, Saudi Arabia and South America.

Diagnosis is confirmed by histology and culture of scrapings and/or biopsy of affected skin (cutaneous form); by light microscopic examination or culture of parasites from splenic or bone marrow aspirates (visceral form). Polymerase chain reaction (PCR) of tissue samples is used to identify the disease-causing species of leishmaniasis, which influences treatment choice.

Treatment is with pentavalent antimonial drugs, meglumine antimoniate (first line) or sodium stibogluconate. Travellers to endemic areas should use insect repellents and appropriate clothing.

Leprosy

Leprosy is a notifiable disease in the UK, caused by *Mycobacterium leprae*, an intracellular bacterium with a predilection for skin, peripheral nerves, respiratory mucosa and eyes. The prevalence is falling, but it is still endemic in India, Africa and South America.

M. leprae causes a chronic granulomatous reaction leading to:
• **Skin:** anaesthetic hypopigmented macules ± erythematous plaques (Figure 22.3a,b).
• **Peripheral nerves:** enlarged peripheral nerves (Figure 22.3a) and peripheral neuropathy.
• **Eyes:** blindness due to direct bacillary infiltration and neuropathy resulting in diminished blinking ± corneal sensation.

It is spread by nasal or oral mucosal droplets from close contact with infected individuals. Incubation period can be up to several years. There are two main subtypes:
1 **Tuberculoid:** strong immune response to *M. leprae*, few skin lesions, low bacterial load (paucibacillary)
2 **Lepromatous:** poor immune response to *M. leprae*, severe disease, with multiple skin lesions and high bacterial load (multibacillary).

Diagnosis is by finding acid-fast bacilli on Ziehl–Neelson staining in smears and/or biopsies from affected skin or other tissue. Serological tests can detect *M. leprae* antigens or antibodies. Treatment is with rifampicin, dapsone and clofazamine, depending on disease subtype. Erythema nodosum leprosum is an immune reaction with red painful skin swelling and fever. It is treated with thalidomide.

Key point

• A skin biopsy helps confirm the diagnosis of leishmaniasis and leprosy.

▶ Warning

• Cutaneous leishmaniasis may progress to mucocutaneous form, leading to mucous membrane destruction.
• Untreated visceral leishmaniasis is potentially fatal.

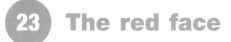

Table 23.1 Specific questions and history

- Where did the eruption start?
- Any history of previous skin disease or family history of skin disease?
- Is this facial eruption itchy?
- Is this facial eruption scaly?
- Any flushing or increased redness (any specific precipitants noted)?
- Any note of allergies or reactions to cosmetics, hair dyes, perfumes?
- Any systemic symptoms such as arthritis or tiredness (anaemia)?

Table 23.3 Specific investigations may be required to confirm diagnosis

- Skin biopsy: histology and direct immunofluorescence (IMF)
- Autoimmune screen: ANA, anti-Ro/La antibodies
- Full blood count, ESR
- Urea and electrolytes, urine analysis
- Serum IgE
- Patch test
- Skin scrapings for mycology

Table 23.2 Causes of a red face and specific examination clues

Rosacea	Papules, pustules and no comedones
Perioral dermatitis	Papules particularly around the mouth
Atopic eczema	Flexural erythema and scaling
Seborrhoeic dermatitis	Scaling, erythema particularly on the eyebrows, nasolabial folds, upper chest and chin
Psoriasis	Well defined scaly patches and plaques on extensor surfaces of limbs and scalp with nail pitting
Contact dermatitis	Vesicles on face occurring after use of particular products
DLE	Diffuse scaling, follicular plugging, atrophy in photosensitive distribution

Fig. 23.1a

Typical rosacea

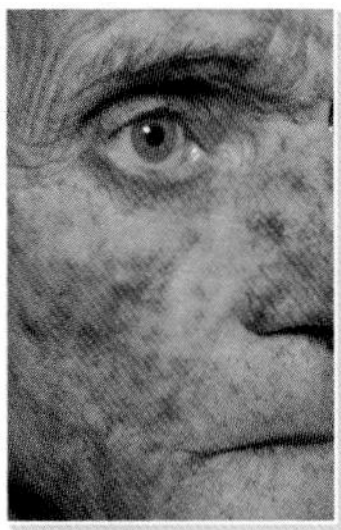

Fig. 23.1b

Note marked telangiectasia

Fig. 23.1c

Note central facial distribution

Fig. 23.1d

Severe rosacea with marked inflammation

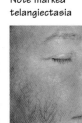
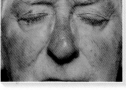
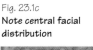
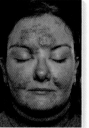

Fig. 23.6a/b

Contact dermatitis to preservatives can affect eyelids

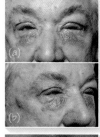

Fig. 23.2a/b

Rhinophyma of nose with distortion of shape – can progress gradually

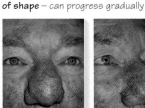
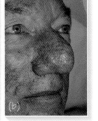

Fig. 23.3a/b **Eczema on face**

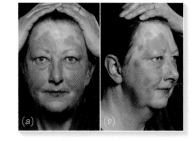

Fig. 23.6c

Contact dermatitis to cosmetic products used on face

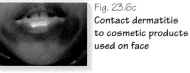

Fig. 23.7a/b

Thick plaques of DLE confirmed on biopsy – this lady later developed SLE

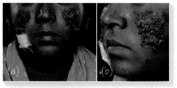

Fig. 23.4

Seborrhoeic dermatitis affecting eyebrows

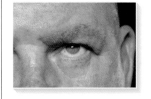

Fig. 23.5a/b **Scaly plaques with sharp borders on scalp margins**

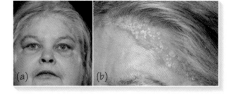

Fig. 23.7c

Telangiectasia and follicular plugging on right cheek

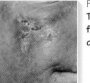

Dermatology at a Glance, First Edition. Mahbub M.U. Chowdhury, Ruwani P. Katugampola, and Andrew Y. Finlay.

It can be difficult to diagnose the cause of a red face. A good knowledge of differential diagnoses is required. Specific history and full skin examination are needed to differentiate conditions such as rosacea, perioral dermatitis, atopic eczema, seborrhoeic dermatitis, psoriasis, contact dermatitis and discoid lupus erythematosus (Tables 23.1–23.3).

Rosacea

Rosacea is a common inflammatory skin disease seen in adults over 30 years old. It is usually confined to the face, mainly affecting the cheeks, forehead, nose and chin. Flushing may occur. Papules, pustules, telangiectasia and erythema are common but no comedones or scaling occur (Figure 23.1). Hypertrophy and lymphoedema of subcutaneous tissue may present with rhinophyma of the nose (Figure 23.2). The cause of rosacea is unknown but it may be triggered by spicy foods and alcohol, leading to flushing and then telangiectasia.

Complications of rosacea include conjunctivitis, keratitis and iritis. Papules and pustules can be treated with antibiotics (topical metronidazole, oral tetracyclines and oral erythromycin) and topical retinoids. Flushing and telangiectasia may not fully respond even to pulse dye laser.

Perioral dermatitis

This is a variant of rosacea that occurs in young females around the mouth or sometimes around the eyes. It usually presents with papules and occasional pustules sparing the skin adjacent to the vermillion border. Other features of rosacea such as flushing and telangiectasia are usually absent. Most cases have a recent history of topical steroid usage. This can improve the eruption but it relapses once the treatment is stopped. Topical steroids need to be stopped and other standard treatments for rosacea such as topical metronidazole and oral antibiotics can be helpful.

Atopic eczema (see Chapter 13)

This can present with facial redness. Eczema can occur on any area of the face with scaling, itching and possible vesicles (Figure 23.3). It is important to take a full history including past and family history of atopy and to examine the whole skin looking for other signs of atopic eczema such as flexural eruption on the limbs. Raised total IgE may help to confirm atopy.

Seborrhoeic dermatitis

This chronic skin condition affects adults with well-defined red scaly patches on the face affecting the eyebrows, nasolabial folds, ears, upper trunk and scalp (Figure 23.4). This condition relapses intermittently and is associated with *Malassezia* yeast. The key feature of seborrhoeic dermatitis is the distribution and usually the rest of the skin is normal with no history of atopy. If severe, immunosuppression such as HIV infection needs to be considered.

Treatment with topical ketoconazole, oral itraconazole, topical steroids (hydrocortisone) and medicated shampoos containing ketoconazole and selenium sulphide.

Psoriasis (see Chapter 12)

Psoriasis commonly affects the face. There may be small patches or plaques particularly along the hairline margin extending from the scalp (Figure 23.5). Patches can be less well defined on the face but signs should be looked for on other areas of the body such as the elbows and knees. The nails can show onycholysis, subungual hyperkeratosis and nail pitting. A family history of psoriasis may also be useful to point towards the correct diagnosis. The eruption is less likely to be severely itchy in psoriasis than in atopic eczema or contact dermatitis.

Contact dermatitis (see Chapter 30)

Irritant contact dermatitis or allergic contact dermatitis may present with facial redness and scaling with or without vesicles (more common with allergy) (Figure 23.6). History taking needs to be targeted towards any specific reactions such as to cosmetics, shampoos, hair dyes or perfumes. There may be a background of consistent reactions to these products and patch testing may be required to differentiate between allergy and irritation.

Discoid lupus erythematosus

Discoid lupus erythematosus (DLE) can present in sun exposed areas particularly on the scalp, face, upper chest and upper trunk (see Chapter 42). The skin shows well-defined erythematous papules and plaques with thickened scaling (Figure 23.7). Typical features of the lesions are central atrophy with scarring, telangiectasia and follicular plugging. The lesions can be either hyperpigmented or depigmented, depending on the skin type. Investigations required are skin biopsy (histology and direct immunofluorescence), autoimmune screen (anti-nuclear antibodies [ANA], anti-Ro/anti-La antibodies), full blood count, erythrocyte sedimentation rate (ESR), urea and electrolytes and urine analysis.

Five per cent of cases progress to systemic lupus erythematosus (SLE). SLE needs to be considered if there are widespread skin lesions and features such as anaemia, reduced white cell count, positive ANA with high titre and arthritis.

Treatment of DLE is sun avoidance and sunscreen use with topical, intralesional or oral corticosteroid therapies. Hydroxychloroquine (anti-malarial), dapsone and systemic retinoids may also be useful.

Tinea faciei

Tinea infection is uncommon on the face but may present with annular scaly patches with central clearing. If topical steroids have been used then the features can be very unusual (tinea incognito). Skin scrapings for mycology are essential to exclude this if suspected.

Key points

- Look for specific pointers in the history and examination to confirm the diagnosis.
- Consider specific tests for SLE and contact allergy.
- Keep an open mind and review the diagnosis if the skin is not improving.

► **Warning**

Topical steroids can worsen rosacea, perioral dermatitis and tinea faciei.

Table 24.1 Approach to a patient with oral and/or genital disease

Clinical history
- Onset, duration, symptoms and functional difficulties due to the genital and/or skin disease
- Skin, nail, hair disease
- Other medical conditions e.g. Crohn's disease
- Current or previous topical treatment/applications to the affected area e.g. scented wipes, over-the-counter creams
- Sexual history where appropriate e.g. high-risk behaviour, previous sexually transmitted infections (STIs)

Clinical examination
- Note the colour, texture of the skin, presence of vesicles, pustules, fissures, ulcers, purpura, discharge, scarring, adhesions of the labia, narrowing of the introitus (females), narrowing of the meatus and difficulty retracting foreskin (males)
- Examine the perineum and peri-anal skin for extension of the genital rash/lesions to these areas
- Examine the whole skin, nails and hair for evidence of associated skin disease

Investigations
- Biopsy affected area if diagnosis uncertain or if non-healing ulcers: histology in all cases, direct immunofluorescence (see Chapter 17) if bullous diseases suspected
- Swab discharge, ulcers, vesicles, pustules for microbiology, virology and STI screen (if appropriate)
- Patch test if allergic contact dermatitis suspected

Table 24.2 Causes and examples of genital skin diseases

- **Inflammatory diseases**
  - lichen sclerosus
  - lichen planus
  - Zoon's balanitis/vulvitis
  - psoriasis
  - eczema (allergic contact dermatitis, lichen simplex)
  - Behçet's disease
  - aphthous ulcers
- **Pigmentary**
  - vitiligo
- **Bullous**
  - bullous pemphigoid
  - pemphigus
- **Pre-malignant**
  - Bowen's disease
- **Malignant**
  - squamous cell carcinoma
  - malignant melanoma
- **Infections**
  - viral e.g. herpes simplex virus, genital warts
  - bacterial e.g. gonorrhoea
  - yeast e.g. candida
  - infestations e.g. scabies (itchy papules)
  - other e.g. syphilis – painless ulcer (primary chancre)
- **Drug-induced**
  - localised ulceration e.g. nicorandil, methotrexate
  - widespread disease e.g. Stevens-Johnson syndrome, toxic epidermal necrolysis

Table 24.3 Causes and examples of oral diseases

- **Inflammatory diseases**
  - lichen planus
  - Behçet's disease
  - aphthous ulcers
- **Pigmentation**
  - benign melanotic macules
  - Addison's disease
- **Bullous**
  - cicatricial pemphigoid
  - pemphigus

- **Infections**
  - viral e.g. herpes simplex virus
  - yeast e.g. candida
  - other e.g. syphilis – characteristic painless 'snail-track' ulcers
- **Drug-induced**
  - localised ulceration e.g. methotrexate
  - widespread disease e.g. Stevens-Johnson syndrome, toxic epidermal necrolysis

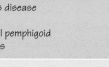

Fig. 24.2
Lichen planus of the buccal mucosa
– note the typical white reticular network (Wickham's striae)

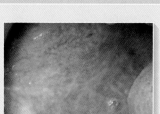

Fig. 24.3
Lichen planus of the gingival mucosa
– the gums may develop painful erosions in erosive lichen planus

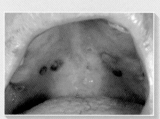

Fig. 24.4
Cicatricial pemphigoid of the palate
– note the haemorrhagic blisters and the subsequent formation of erosions

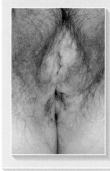

Fig 24.1
Lichen sclerosus of the vulva and peri-anal skin
– note the pallor and haemorrhagic purpura in the figure-of-eight distribution affecting the vulva and peri-anal skin

Genital and oral mucosal diseases may be localised or be part of a generalised skin disease (e.g. lichen planus).

Genital skin disease

Inflammatory genital skin diseases

Psoriasis presents with symmetrical well-demarcated erythematous shiny plaques which lack the typical scales.

Eczema has ill-defined itchy erythematous patches, with hyperpigmentation and lichenification due to chronic scratching.

Lichen sclerosus (LS) commonly presents in pre-pubertal and post-menopausal females with itchy and/or painful erythema, fissures and erosions of the vulval and peri-anal skin leading to scarring. Atrophic skin with purpura is seen in its quiescent phase (Figure 24.1). In men, similar features are seen on the glans penis. Complications include narrowing of the vaginal introitus, labial adhesions in females, phimosis in males and urethral strictures.

Lichen planus (LP) presents with itchy shiny violaceous papules, plaques or erosions on the vulva, shaft or glans penis.

Zoon's balanitis or vulvitis, also called plasma cell balanitis or vulvitis based on its histological features, presents with asymptomatic red shiny plaques on the glans penis or vulva.

Management

- Patients should be examined with sensitivity and due respect.
- Table 24.1 summarises the clinical approach and investigations.
- Avoid irritant and fragranced products (e.g. scented wipes).
- Use bland emollients as soap substitutes and moisturisers.
- Genital psoriasis, eczema and Zoon's balanitis/vulvitis generally respond to a few weeks' treatment with mild to moderately potent topical corticosteroids.
- LS and LP require super-potent topical corticosteroids, initially once daily for a month, then alternate days for a further month followed by 2–3 times per week as required.
- LS or LP unresponsive to topical therapy may require systemic treatment (e.g. methotrexate, acitretin).
- Circumcision can be curative for Zoon's balanitis.
- There is a <5% risk of malignancy developing within LS in women; the risk is less in men.

Infectious genital skin diseases

Genital warts are caused by the human papilloma virus (HPV). They present with small warty papules or larger lesions on the penis, vulva and perineum, and may extend to the cervix and/or rectum. HPV types 16 and 18 are associated with pre-malignant and malignant transformation of the genital skin. Treatment includes topical 5% imiquimod cream. Topical podophyllin and cryotherapy are also used.

Pubic or crab lice are caused by *Phthirus pubis* and transmitted by person-to-person body contact. The female louse lays eggs around the pubic hair shafts, which hatch a week later. Presentation is with itchy red papules in the pubic area. Treatment is as for scabies (see Chapter 21).

Herpes simplex virus (HSV) infection presents with tingling sensation followed by development of grouped vesicles, ulceration, crusting and healing. Genital HSV is contagious and spreads by direct contact. Treatment is topical and/or oral aciclovir.

Syphilis is caused by the spirochete, *Treponema pallidum*, and acquired as a sexually transmitted infection (STI). Initial presentation is with a painless genital ulcer (primary chancre) associated with inguinal lymphadenopathy 2 weeks after acquiring the infection. Syphilis serology may not become positive during the appearance of the primary chancre. The spirochetes may be visible on dark field microscopy of the ulcer fluid. The ulcer resolves spontaneously. Secondary syphilis will follow 1–3 months after the primary chancre characterised by an asymptomatic papular rash with collarette of scale on the palms, soles of the feet and trunk. Parenteral penicillin is the treatment of choice (doses and duration vary according to stage of disease).

Oral mucosal disease (Figures 24.2–24.4)

Lichen planus presents as a white net-like reticular pattern (Wickham's striae) and erosions on the buccal and gingival mucosa.

Aphthous ulcers are the most common type of mouth ulcers. These painful ulcers are well demarcated with a yellowish centre and erythematous edge. They occur as an isolated episode or may recur, precipitated by stress and trauma.

Behçet's disease is a chronic multi-system vasculitis leading to recurrent oral and genital ulcers, arthritis and skin lesions (e.g. erythema nodosum).

Cicatricial pemphigoid (mucous membrane pemphigoid) presents with blisters of the oral and/or ocular mucosa, leading to erosions and scarring. Other mucosal and skin surfaces may be involved (e.g. oesophagus, nasal and genital mucosa, scalp skin).

Management

- Potent to super-potent topical corticosteroids, in ointment form for better mucosal adhesion. Oral LP and aphthous ulcers can also be treated with hydrocortisone oral mucosal pellets held in contact with lesions. Steroid inhalers (e.g. beclometasone) can be sprayed on to gingival LP.
- Anaesthetics (e.g. lidocaine gel) can be used for pain relief.
- Cicatricial pemphigoid affecting the eyes and oesophagus requires early intervention to prevent scarring and associated complications of visual impairment and dysphagia. Use systemic steroids with azathioprine or intravenous cyclophosphomide.
- Oral colchicine, dapsone and thalidomide have been effective in managing the systemic manifestations of Behçet's disease.

Key points

- Differential diagnosis of recurrent mouth and/or genital ulcers include Behçet's disease, cicatricial pemphigoid, pemphigus, infections (e.g. syphilis) or drug-induced causes.
- Sexual contacts of those with STIs should be traced and treated.

▶ **Warning**

Non-healing oral and/or genital ulcers and lesions should be biopsied to exclude pre-malignant or malignant disease.

Table 25.1 Approach to a patient with nail/or hair disease

Clinical history
- Underlying skin disease
- Underlying systemic diseases
- Menstrual history, e.g. amenorrhoea or irregular periods in polycystic ovarian syndrome associated with hirsutism, heavy periods resulting in iron deficiency, diffuse non-scarring alopecia and koilonychia
- Current and relevant previous medication and treatment, e.g. radiotherapy for ring worm infection (pre-1940s) or skin cancer resulting in localised scarring alopecia of the scalp

Clinical examination
- Examine all 20 nails, taking note of their shape, colour, texture and surface changes
- Examine the scalp skin for evidence of scarring, erythema and scaling, texture and strength of hair shaft, distribution and volume of hair
- Distribution of hair in other parts of the body, e.g. face, limbs, axillae
- Examine the whole skin including oral mucosa for associated skin disease
- Physical examination for evidence of underlying disease, e.g. cardiac disease (clubbing of nails), virilisation (hirsute woman)

Investigations
- Nail clippings and scalp skin scraping for mycology (fungal nail infections or tinea capitis)
- Nail biopsy (subungual melanoma)
- Microscopy for hair shaft abnormalities (bamboo-shaped hair in Netherton's syndrome)
- Serum ferritin (koilonychia & diffuse non-scarring alopecia)
- Serum luteinising & follicular stimulating hormones, testosterone, androstenedione (hirsutism), thyroid function (diffuse alopecia, alopecia areata)
- Ultrasound scan of pelvis (polycystic ovaries)
- Other: porphyria screen, pituitary hormone profile

Table 25.2 Causes and examples of nail disease

Pitting
- Psoriasis, lichen planus, alopecia areata

Subungual hyperkeratosis
- Psoriasis, fungal infections, viral warts, squamous cell carcinoma

Onycholysis
- Psoriasis, fungal infections

Longitudinal ridging of nail plate
- Darier's disease, lichen planus

Shape of nail plate
- Koilonychia e.g. iron deficiency
- Clubbing e.g. cystic fibrosis, endocarditis

Colour changes of the nail
- **Black** e.g. racial melanonychia, subungual haematoma, melanoma
- **Yellow** e.g. yellow nail syndrome, jaundice
- **White** e.g. chronic renal failure, hypoalbuminaemia

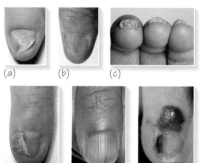

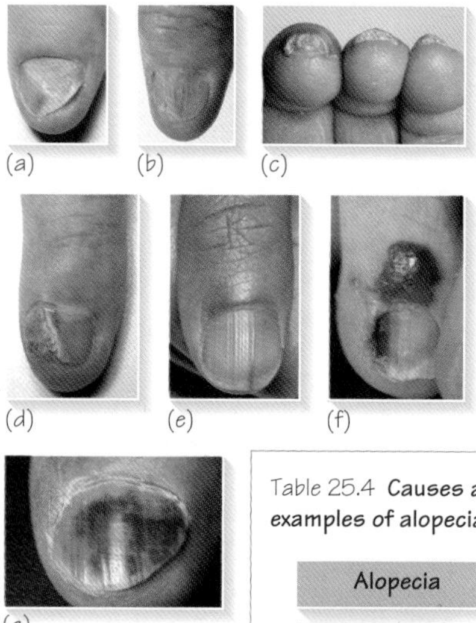

Fig 25.1a–g Clinical images of nail disease
(a) **Nail psoriasis:** Note the pitting of the proximal nail plate and onycholysis of the distal nail plate
(b) **Lichen planus affecting the nail:** Note the longitudinal ridging of the nail plate and adhesions between the posterior nailfold and nail plate (pterygium)
(c) **Subungual hyperkeratosis**
(d) **Subungual viral wart affecting nail growth**
(e) **Longitudinal melanonychia:** Normal finding in racially pigmented individuals
(f) **Subungual melanoma:** Note the pigmentation of the surrounding skin due to the melanoma (Hutchinson's sign)
(g) **Subungual haematoma:** Note the normal cuticle

Table 25.3 Causes and examples of diseases leading to excess hair growth

Excess hair

Hirsutism
- Endogenous androgens, e.g. polycystic ovary syndrome, androgen-secreting ovarian or adrenal tumours
- Pituitary disorders, e.g. Cushing's disease
- Medication, e.g. long-term systemic steroids

Hypertrichosis
- Medication, e.g. minoxidil, ciclosporin
- Systemic diseases, e.g. porphyria cutanea tarda

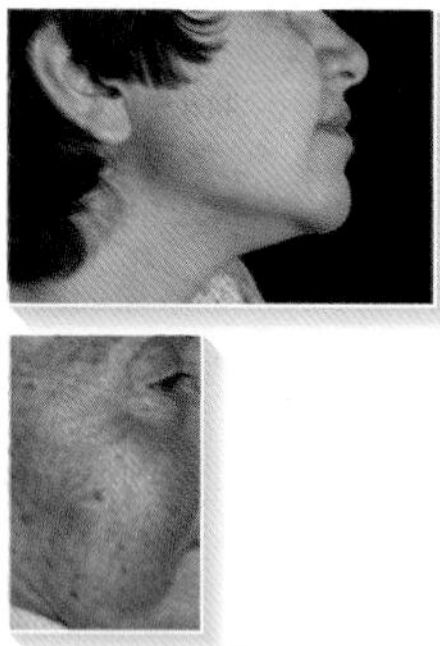

Fig 25.3a/b Clinical images of excess hair
(a) **Hirsutism:** Dark coarse shaven hair in the beard distribution on face in a female with polycystic ovary syndrome
(b) **Hypertrichosis:** Diffuse fine hair on the face of a patient with porphyria cutanea tarda

Table 25.4 Causes and examples of alopecia

Alopecia

Non-scarring
- Telogen effluvium
- Androgenetic alopecia
- Alopecia areata
- Self-induced (trichotillomania)
- Inflammatory, e.g. psoriasis
- Hair shaft disorders, e.g. bamboo shaped hair (trichorrhexis invaginata) in Netherton's syndrome
- Drug-induced, e.g. warfarin, retinoids
- Infections, e.g. tinea capitis
- Systemic diseases, e.g. hypothyroidism, iron-deficiency

Scarring
- Inflammatory skin diseases, e.g. lichen planus, lupus erythematosus, folliculitis decalvans
- Neoplastic, e.g. basal cell carcinoma
- Treatment-related, e.g. radiotherapy

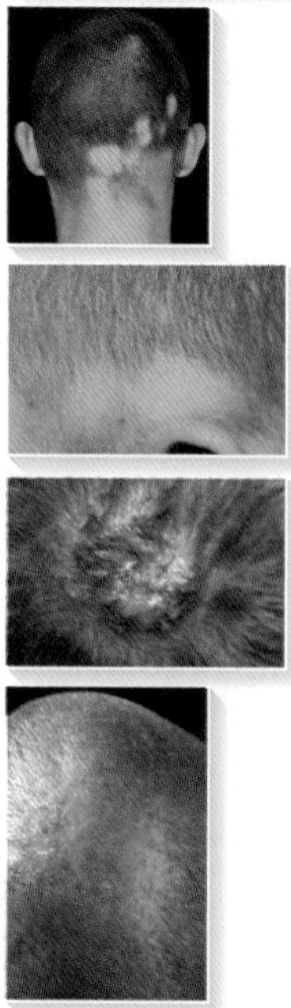

Fig 25.4a–d Clinical images of alopecia
(a) **Alopecia areata**
(b) **Alopecia areata** (closeup view): Note the regrowth of short hairs within the patches of alopecia
(c) **Scaly plaque on the scalp with underlying inflammation:** The differential diagnosis includes psoriasis, tinea capitis
(d) **Scarring alopecia of the scalp:** The underlying condition in this patient was previously treated folliculitis decalvans

Hair and nail diseases are congenital or acquired. They may be seen in isolation and independent of each other or associated with skin or systemic disease (e.g. lichen planus of the skin, nails and scarring alopecia). A systematic approach to nail and hair diseases will help identify the cause and aid treatment (Table 25.1).

Nail diseases

Different presentations, causes and examples of nail diseases are summarised in Table 25.2. Trauma is by far the most common cause of a black or red subungual lesion, but **subungual melanoma** should be considered in subungual hyperpigmentation. A diagnostic clue is the (often variable) pigmentation of the posterior nail fold (Hutchinson's sign). A longitudinal nail biopsy will confirm the diagnosis. The whole lesion should be surgically excised with adequate surgical margins. The patient should be followed up regularly for monitoring of recurrence or metastatic disease.

Management

• Fungal nail infections require 3–4 months of oral anti-fungal treatment with terbinafine or itraconazole.
• Specific treatment of nail changes due to skin or systemic diseases are difficult. Systemic treatment given for the underlying skin disease may improve the nail changes (e.g. methotrexate or biological treatments for psoriasis).
• General practical management advice includes keeping nails cut short and moisturised to reduce trauma and breakage of nails. In onycholysis, nail lacquer may improve the cosmetic appearance.

Hair

The human skin has three types of hair. Fine, soft, fair **lanugo hair** covers most of the fetus's skin *in utero* and is shed prior to a full-term birth. Fine **vellous hair** develops on most of the skin after birth, except for the palms and soles of feet. Coarse, darker **terminal hairs** occur on the scalp. During puberty, terminal hairs also develop in the axillae, pubic area and beard area in men.

Each human hair goes through a cycle: active growth phase (**anagen**), which may last a few years, followed by cessation of cell division in the hair bulb (**catagen**) and hair shedding (**telogen**) (see Chapter 4).

Excess hair

Hirsutism is increased growth of terminal hair in women in a male pattern distribution. **Hypertrichosis** is increased growth of terminal hair in a non-male distribution, which may be localised or generalised. Causes, examples and investigation of hirsutism and hypertrichosis are summarised in Tables 25.1 and 25.3.

In addition to treatment of the underlying cause, the following are aimed at decreasing excess hair: plucking, shaving, waxing, electrolysis, topical eflornithine (slows the rate of hair growth by inhibiting ornithine decarboxylase), laser, systemic anti-androgen for hirsutism due to polycystic ovary syndrome (e.g. Dianette®).

Alopecia

Hair loss may be localised or diffuse, scarring or non-scarring. Causes, examples and investigation of alopecia are summarised in Tables 25.4 and 25.1.

Telogen effluvium

This is diffuse sudden hair loss a few months after a significant illness or pregnancy. Explanation and reassurance of hair regrowth in a few months is all that is required.

Male pattern hair loss (androgenetic alopecia)

This is common in men, but also occurs in women. There is often a family history of male pattern alopecia. The scalp skin is normal. The common hair loss patterns are the frontal–temporal region and vertex (men and women) and diffuse hair loss sparing the parietal and occipital scalp (usually men). Exclude other causes of diffuse hair loss (Table 25.4).

Treatment: topical minoxidil (2% for women, 5% for men), oral finasteride (for men) and hair transplant (specialist centres).

Alopecia areata

The aetiology is unknown but possibly due to autoimmune destruction of hair follicles. There may be a personal or family history of other autoimmune diseases such as Hashimoto's thyroiditis or vitiligo.

Presentation and progression can range from a single or several round patches of hair loss on normal scalp skin to complete hair loss on the scalp (totalis) or whole body (universalis). Hair may regrow spontaneously (initially depigmented). Poor prognostic features include childhood onset, alopecia totalis or universalis and presence of exclamation mark hairs (short hairs that are dark distally, and thin and depigmented towards the scalp) suggesting continuing disease activity.

Treatment: topical or intralesional steroids, topical irritants (dithranol) and sensitizers (dinitrochlorobenzene), phototherapy (PUVA) and, rarely, oral steroids or immunosuppression with oral ciclosporin.

Alopecia associated with inflammatory skin diseases

Psoriasis and eczema cause localised or diffuse non-scarring alopecia with erythema of the scalp. As there is no scarring, the prognosis for hair regrowth is good once the disease has been treated.

Local treatment for psoriasis and eczema of the scalp includes topical steroid application, the topical vitamin D analogue calcipotriol (psoriasis only) and tar-based shampoo.

Discoid lupus erythematosus and lichen planus can affect the scalp resulting in scarring, destruction of the hair follicles and permanent hair loss. In addition to systemic treatment (see Chapter 42), local treatment includes potent topical corticosteroids to control the inflammation.

Key points

• Consider an underlying systemic cause for nail or hair diseases.
• Spontaneous hair regrowth is common in alopecia areata; poor prognostic factors predict progression of alopecia.

▶ **Warning**

Subungual melanoma should be considered if subungual hyperpigmentation is present.

Table 26.1   Skin manifestations of the newborn

- **Benign physiological phenomenon & skin pigmentation** e.g. cutis marmorata, mongolian blue spots
- **Transient rashes** e.g. neonatal acne, miliaria, toxic erythema of the newborn, transient neonatal pustular melanosis
- **Persistent and/or progressive rashes or skin diseases**
  - hereditary: epidermolysis bullosa, disorders of keratinisation (e.g. ichthyosis vulgaris)
  - acquired: inflammatory (e.g. seborrhoeic dermatitis, atopic eczema), trans-placental transfer of maternal auto-antibodies (e.g. neonatal lupus erythematosus)
- **Skin lesions**
  - vascular malformation, haemangioma
  - melanocytic naevi

Fig. 26.1   **Cutis marmorata**

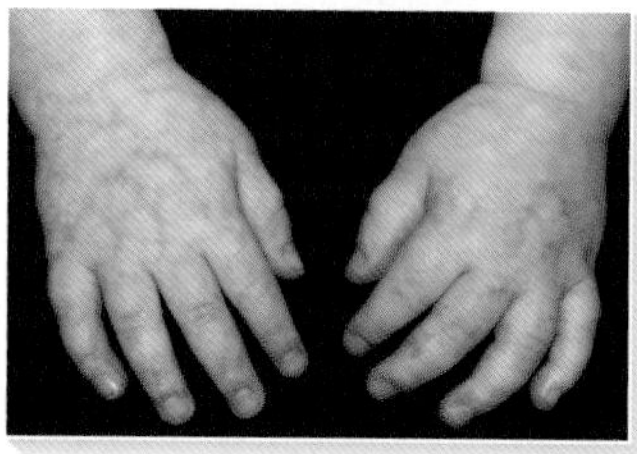

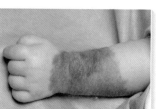

Fig. 26.2   **Mongolian blue spot on the lower back**

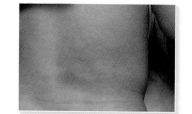

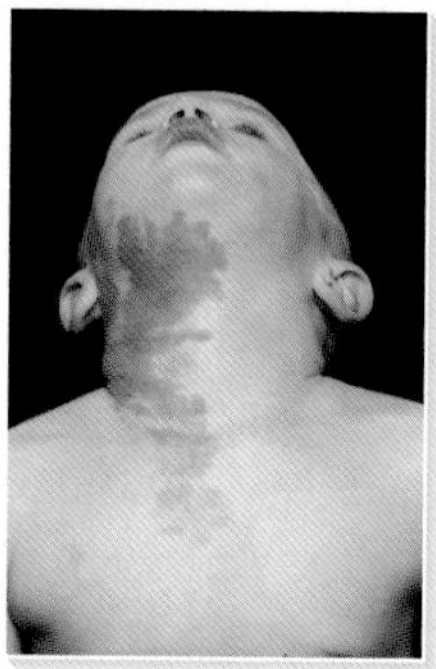

Fig. 26.3 **Vascular malformation** (port wine stain)

Fig. 26.4   **An infantile haemangioma**

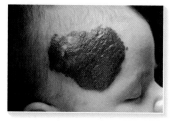

Fig. 26.5   **A regressing infantile haemangioma**

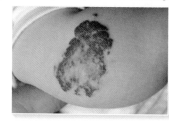

Fig. 26.6 **Ulcerated large haemangioma on the arm**

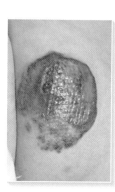

Fig. 26.7 **Congenital melanocytic naevus** – note the hair and variable pigmentation within the naevus

Table 26.2   Differentiating features between vascular malformations and infantile haemangiomas

	Vascular malformation	Infantile haemangioma
Onset	Present at birth	Within the first few weeks/months of life
Clinical course	Grows with the child (does not regress)	Rapid proliferation in the first few months followed by spontaneous regression over years
Histological features	Combination of one or more of mature capillary, arterial, venous and lymphatic channels	Endothelial hyperplasia (proliferative phase) followed by fibrosis (regression phase)

The skin of newborn infants may be covered by vernix caseosa, a white lipid-containing material. The skin barrier function is normal at full-term birth, but impaired if premature. Table 26.1 lists skin conditions seen in newborn infants.

▶ **Warning**

Skin barrier function is impaired in premature neonates, so increased risk systemic absorption of topical steroids.

Dermatology at a Glance, First Edition. Mahbub M.U. Chowdhury, Ruwani P. Katugampola, and Andrew Y. Finlay.

Benign physiological phenomenon

Cutis marmorata is a transient, net-like mottled violaceous discoloration caused by a normal physiological response to a cool environment (Figure 26.1). Persistent cutis marmorata may be associated with limb hypertrophy and macrocephaly.

Benign skin pigmentation

Mongolian blue spots are slate-grey to blue flat patches on the lower back or buttocks in neonates of Asian, Oriental or Afro-Caribbean origin (Figure 26.2). They are benign and disappear with time.

Transient rashes

Neonatal acne

Infants present with papules and pustules on the cheeks which resolve after a few months. The condition results from stimulation of neonatal sebaceous glands by trans-placental transfer of maternal adrenal androgens. Acne cysts may develop, requiring systemic antibiotics such as erythromycin to prevent scarring.

Miliaria

Miliaria are multiple clear to yellowish vesicles seen on the face of neonates, especially in warm and humid environments, caused by blocked and/or immature sweat ducts. They resolve spontaneously.

Toxic erythema of the newborn

This is an erythematous macular rash with yellow papules containing eosinophils. It occurs on the face, trunk and limbs in the first few days of life and resolves spontaneously over a few days.

Transient neonatal pustular melanosis

This is an asymptomatic rash of unknown aetiology which appears on the first day of life. It consists of vesicles and pustules on the trunk, palms and soles which then rupture to form pigmented macules. It resolves spontaneously over a few months.

Persistent and/or progressive rashes

Seborrhoeic dermatitis

One of the most common, often self-limiting skin diseases seen in infants. The exact cause is unknown.

Infants present with an asymptomatic, red, ill-defined scaly rash affecting the scalp ('cradle cap'), face and napkin area including skin folds (in contrast to napkin dermatitis, which spares skin folds).

Treatment: emollients and mild steroids (e.g. 1% hydrocortisone) to control inflammation and olive oil to loosen scalp scaling.

Neonatal lupus erythematosus

Infants present with erythematous scaly macules and plaques on the face and trunk which resolve spontaneously within months. Caused by trans-placental transfer of maternal auto-antibodies (anti-Ro antibodies) which can lead to congenital heart block. Management of the skin includes photoprotection and topical mild corticosteroids. Heart block requires cardiology care and possible pacemaker.

Skin lesions

Table 26.2 summarises the differentiating features between vascular malformations and infantile haemangiomas.

Vascular malformations

These vary in size, can occur anywhere on the body and be cosmetically distressing for children and parents (Figure 26.3). They are initially flat, but become raised and darker with age.

Treatment: pulsed dye laser, cosmetic camouflage.
Complications: glaucoma, if overlying an eye.

- **Naevus flammeus:** flat pink telangiectatic mark seen in up to 50% of newborn infants on the back of the neck ('stork mark') or forehead ('angel's kiss'). Usually fades with time.
- **Sturge–Weber syndrome:** capillary malformation (port-wine stain) in segment(s) of the trigeminal nerve distribution with underlying intra-cranial angiomas associated with epilepsy.
- **Klippel–Trénaunay syndrome:** triad of vascular malformation of a limb associated with venous varicosities and overgrowth of the underlying soft tissues and bone.

Infantile haemangiomas

The most common benign tumours of infancy. Vary in size, body site and number and appear as well-demarcated bright red plaques or nodules during the proliferative stage (Figure 26.4). When regressing, the lesions flatten and become purple and grey (Figure 26.5). Haemangiomas regress spontaneously: about 50% by 5 years of age, and the remainder by 10 years. Most do not require treatment unless they develop complications or interfere with function (e.g. haemangioma on the lip or ano-genital region).

Complications: bleeding, ulceration, infection (Figure 26.6).

Treatment: bleeding can be controlled with direct pressure. Ulcerated haemangiomas require wound care, analgesia, topical and/or oral antibiotics and pulsed dye laser. Systemic propranolol is effective for large, rapidly proliferating haemangiomas. Infants with >5 (or rarely hundreds) haemangiomas may have extracutaneous haemangiomas in one or more of the following: liver, heart, brain, gastrointestinal tract or eyes. Depending on the organs involved, the infant is at risk of potential life-threatening haemorrhage and must be managed by a specialist multi-disciplinary team.

Congenital melanocytic naevi (Figure 26.7)

Present at birth and vary in size from a few millimetres to several centimetres across. Often deeply pigmented, usually flat but may be palpable, contain terminal hair and show colour variation. Giant naevi (>20 cm diameter) may have surrounding multiple smaller satellite naevi.

Complications of giant congenital naevi: cosmetic issues, risk of malignant transformation to melanoma at a young age. Naevi overlying the head, neck and spine may rarely be associated with melanosis of the meninges and central nervous system and neurophysiological abnormalities.

Management: monitor naevi with serial photographs, excise suspicious areas, large naevi may require multi-step surgery with use of tissue expanders and skin grafts. If naevi overlying the head, neck and spine in infants a practical approach is for regular neurological examination with magnetic resonance imaging.

Key points

- Vascular malformations in trigeminal distribution may have glaucoma and intra-cranial complications.
- Giant congenital melanocytic naevi are associated with a small but significant risk of malignant melanoma.
- Most infantile haemangiomas regress spontaneously and do not require intervention unless complications.

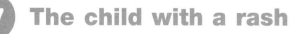

27 The child with a rash

Table 27.1 **Approach to a child with a rash**

Clinical history	Clinical examination	Investigations
• Onset: acute or chronic • Systemic symptoms (fever) • Duration of rash • Change in rash over time (intermittent, progressive) • Symptoms of rash (itching, pain) • Family history of skin disease • Recent contact with individuals with a rash (scabies, chickenpox) • Drug history • Other medical history (atopy: asthma, hay fever) • Other history: insect bites, contact with plants	• Distribution of the rash (generalised, localised, extensor or flexor aspects of limbs) • Morphology of the rash/lesions (see Table 27.2) • Involvement of nails, scalp, mucosal surfaces (e.g. tinea corporis and psoriasis may both involve the nails and scalp) • Systemic manifestations (fever in infectious causes)	• Skin scrapings for mycology • Swab for microbiology (e.g. impetigo) • Skin biopsy (blistering rashes or when diagnosis uncertain) • Blood investigations depending on diagnosis: blood cultures (bacterial meningitis), viral serology, full blood count, coagulation screen, renal function for purpuric/petechial rashes • Blood pressure and urine dipstick for evidence of haematuria in purpuric/petechial rashes

Table 27.2 **Clues to diagnosis based on the morphology of the rash in a child**

- **Macular (+/− papular) rash** – viral exanthem (e.g. measles, rubella), drug-induced (e.g. penicillin, phenytoin), Kawasaki disease
- **Papular rash** – scabies, molluscum contagiosum
- **Papulovesicular rash** – chickenpox
- **Scaly rash** – eczema, psoriasis, tinea corporis, pityriasis versicolor, pityriasis rosea
- **Blistering rash** – insect bites, bullous impetigo, linear IgA bullous disease, epidermolysis bullosa, staphylococcal scalded skin syndrome, Stevens-Johnson syndrome/toxic epidermal necrolysis
- **Urticarial rash** – idiopathic urticaria, urticaria pigmentosa
- **Petechial/purpuric rash** – meningococcal septicaemia, Henoch–Schönlein purpura, haemorrhagic oedema of infancy, haematological disease (leukaemia, idiopathic thrombocytopaenic purpura), non-accidental injury

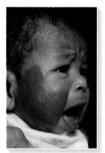
Fig. 27.1 **Atopic eczema**

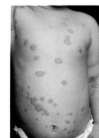
Fig. 27.2 **Psoriasis**

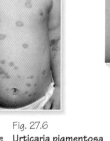
Fig. 27.3 **Molluscum contagiosum**

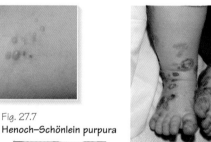
Fig. 27.4 **Linear IgA bullous disease** – note the distribution of blisters in an arc-like pattern

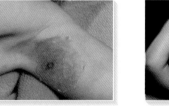
Fig. 27.5 **Staphylococcal scalded skin syndrome**

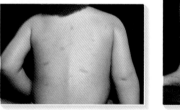
Fig. 27.6 **Urticaria pigmentosa**

Fig. 27.7 **Henoch–Schönlein purpura**

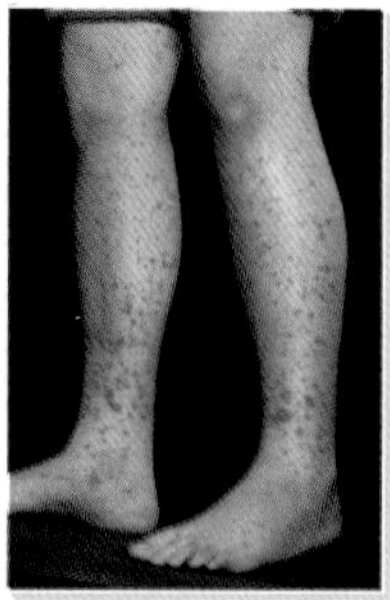

There are many causes of children's rashes (Tables 27.1 and 27.2). The papular rash scabies is described in Chapter 21. The scaly rashes atopic eczema and psoriasis (Figures 27.1 and 27.2) are described in Chapters 12 and 13. Urticaria is described in Chapter 32. For the blistering rashes, bullous impetigo see Chapter 18 and epidermolysis bullosa see Chapter 46.

> **Warning**
>
> A febrile child with a non-blanching petechial and/or purpuric rash should be treated promptly with systemic antibiotics for presumed meningococcal septicaemia.

Macular (± papular) rash

Measles presents as an erythematous maculopapular rash starting on the face, spreads to the trunk and fades over a few days. Koplik's spots (transient clusters of white papules with red halo) on the buccal mucosa, fever, cough and lymphadenopathy occur. Incidence of measles in the UK has risen because of some children missing their measles, mumps and rubella (MMR) vaccination. Treatment is symptomatic with monitoring for complications (e.g. pneumonia). Diagnosis is clinical but viral DNA may be identified on blood culture.

Papular rash

Molluscum contagiosum (Figure 27.3) is a common poxvirus infection. Skin-coloured papules with central umbilication develop on the trunk, face or limbs. Lesions are self-limiting but treatments include cryotherapy, curettage or topical 5% imiquimod cream.

Papular–vesicular rash

Chickenpox is a highly contagious airborne disease caused by varicella zoster virus. Patients present with general malaise, fever and an itchy papular–vesicular rash on the head and trunk; lesions heal over a week with or without scarring. Diagnosis is usually clinical. Treatment is symptomatic with monitoring for complications (e.g. pneumonia); antiviral treatment (e.g. aciclovir) started within 48 hours of the rash onset may decrease the disease severity. Reactivation of the varicella zoster virus causes shingles (herpes zoster).

Blistering rash

Linear IgA bullous disease (chronic bullous disease of childhood)

This is caused by IgA autoantibodies against the bullous pemphigoid antigen on the basement membrane. Blisters develop in an arc pattern (Figure 27.4) and may occur in the mouth and eyes. Skin biopsy shows a subepidermal blister; direct immunofluorescence of peri-lesion skin shows linear IgA deposition along the epidermal basement membrane. The disease resolves over a few years, but may recur.

Treatment: topical steroids and oral steroids with dapsone.

Staphylococcal scalded skin syndrome

Staphylococcal scalded skin syndrome (SSSS) is caused by disruption of epidermal keratinocyte adhesion by circulating exfoliative toxins produced by specific phage-types of *Staphylococcus aureus*.

The child presents with pyrexia and tender erythema followed by superficial blistering, desquamation and re-epithelialisation over 2 weeks (Figure 27.5). Flexures are often affected.

Investigations: swab possible sources of primary *Staphylococcus aureus* infection (nose, throat, skin) for culture and sensitivity, blood cultures, full blood count (FBC) and renal function.

Management: analgesia, systemic flucloxacillin, emollients, non-adherent dressings for eroded skin, pressure-relieving mattress to minimise friction and skin blistering. Diagnosis is clinical but a skin biopsy may be required to exclude other diagnoses (e.g. Stevens–Johnson syndrome and toxic epidermal necrolysis; see Chapter 16). Mucosal surfaces are spared in SSSS and there is no epidermal necrosis on skin biopsy.

Urticarial rash

Urticaria pigmentosa

Urticaria pigmentosa (UP) is a cutaneous mastocytosis caused by increased mast cells. Multiple brown macules are seen, with or without papules, often on the trunk (Figure 27.6). Lesions itch and urticate when rubbed (Darier's sign), or if the child is active or warm. Mutations in *c-kit* gene can cause UP.

Management: oral anti-histamines and avoiding triggers that may result in massive release of histamine such as physical triggers (heat, vigorous rubbing, exertion), medication (aspirin, non-steroidal anti-inflammatory drugs, codeine, morphine), radiocontrast media and some general anaesthetics. It resolves spontaneously by adulthood in about 50% of children. If lymphadenopathy with or without hepato-splenomegaly investigate for **systemic mastocytosis** (rare in childhood).

Petechial and purpuric rash

These result from disorders of blood vessels (e.g. vasculitis) or blood (e.g. idiopathic thrombocytopenic purpura, leukaemia).

Henoch–Schönlein purpura

This is a self-limiting, IgA-mediated vasculitis associated with preceding infection (e.g. streptococcal upper respiratory tract infection). Characterised by a palpable purpuric rash of buttocks and lower legs, with some necrotic and ulcerated lesions, and resolving over 1 month (Figure 27.7). The vasculitis may affect the kidney and/or gastrointestinal tract.

Investigations: throat swabs, serum anti-streptolysin O titres, ESR, CRP, FBC, serum electrolytes, urea and creatinine, urine for haematuria, proteinuria and blood pressure. Skin biopsy is rarely needed, as the diagnosis is clinical.

Treatment: non-steroidal anti-inflammatory analgesia, rest and penicillin (if streptococcal infection). Renal involvement determines prognosis and may need systemic steroids.

Important conditions not to miss

Meningococcal septicaemia

The child develops flu-like symptoms, high fever, headache, neck stiffness and a widespread macular erythematous rash that changes into petechiae with or without purpura. The petechiae do not blanch when a glass tumbler is pressed on the skin. There may be rapid progression to septicaemic shock with brain damage or death. Suspected meningococcal septicaemia should be treated with intravenous or intramuscular benzylpenicillin or cefotaxime immediately.

Kawasaki's disease

An acute multi-system vasculitic disease that usually affects children aged under 5 years. It is characterised by fever for at least 5 days, cervical lymphadenopathy, conjunctival injection, strawberry tongue, red fissured lips, maculopapular rash, oedema, erythema and desquamation of hands and feet. Prompt management is essential to prevent complications (e.g. myocardial infarction).

Investigations: FBC, ESR, CRP, ECG, echocardiography, angiography and CT (to detect coronary aneurysms).

Treatment: intravenous immunoglobulins with high-dose aspirin until resolution of inflammatory markers and cardiac complications.

> ### Key points
>
> - In urticaria pigmentosa avoid trigger factors that risk massive endogenous histamine release and shock.
> - Treat suspected Kawasaki's disease promptly with intravenous immunoglobulins and high-dose aspirin to minimise cardiovascular complications.

Table 28.1 **Skin problems in pregnancy**

Physiological skin changes in pregnancy

- Increased pigmentation e.g. areola of breast, melasma (usually face)
- Spider naevi (commonly chest wall)
- Striae on the abdominal wall
- Diffuse non-scarring alopecia post-partum with subsequent normal regrowth of hair (telogen effluvium)

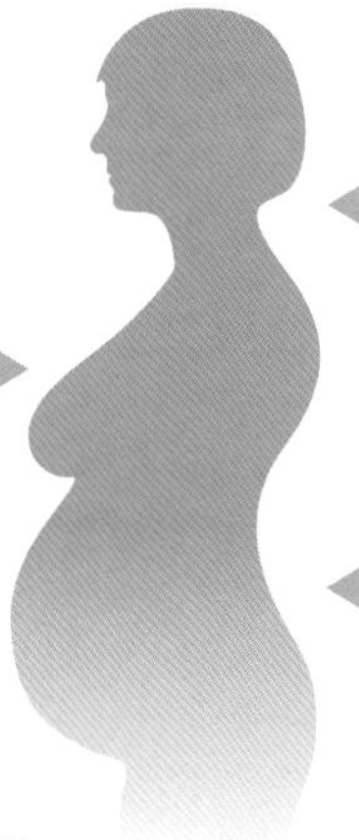

Pregnancy-related dermatoses

- Intra-hepatic cholestasis of pregnancy
- Polymorphic eruption of pregnancy
- Pemphigoid gestationis

Skin lesions in pregnancy

- Benign skin tags
- Thickening or increased pigmentation of pre-existing melanocytic naevi
- Pyogenic granuloma
- Malignant melanoma

Table 28.2 **Differentiation between pregnancy-related dermatoses**

Characteristic features	Intra-hepatic cholestasis of pregnancy	Polymorphic eruption of pregnancy*	Pemphigoid gestationis
Clinical features	Severe generalised itching +/− jaundice	Extremely itchy urticated papules and plaques	Extremely itchy blistering eruption
Characteristic distribution	Mainly palms and soles of feet	Abdominal wall with peri-umbilical sparing	Widespread, including peri-umbilical area
Risk to fetus	Fetal distress, prematurity, stillbirth	None	Small for dates fetus
Prognosis	Could recur in subsequent pregnancies or in association with oral contraceptive pill	Usually does not recur in subsequent pregnancies; less severe if recurs	Recurs more severely in subsequent pregnancies, menstrual cycle or with oral contraceptive pill

*Also termed Pruritic Urticated Papules and Plaques of Pregnancy (PUPPP)

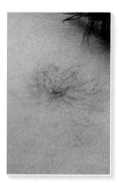

Fig. 28.1
Spider naevus
– benign telangiectasia with a central arteriole that blanches on pressure. Seen in children, pregnant women and multiple lesions in association with liver disease

Fig. 28.2
Melasma on the face
– hyperpigmentation, commonly seen on the face, in association with high oestrogen states (e.g. pregnancy, use of the oral contraceptive pill)

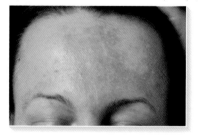

Fig. 28.3 **Benign skin tags**

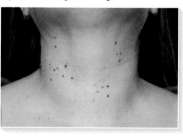

Fig. 28.4 **Pyogenic granuloma**

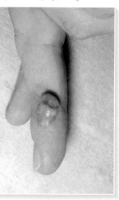

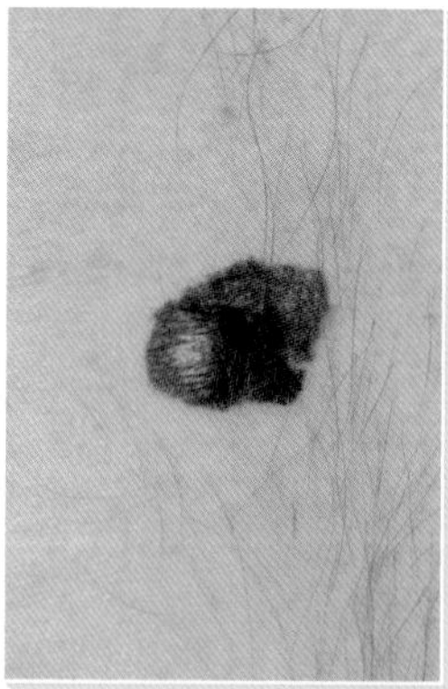

Fig. 28.5
Malignant melanoma

Fig. 28.6
Polymorphic eruption of pregnancy
– note the characteristic peri-umbilical sparing

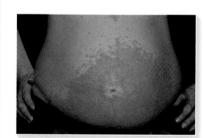

Dermatology at a Glance, First Edition. Mahbub M.U. Chowdhury, Ruwani P. Katugampola, and Andrew Y. Finlay.

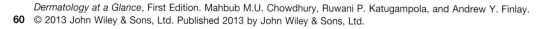

Physiological skin changes in pregnancy

Physiological skin changes occur in women during pregnancy (Table 28.1). Patients require reassurance regarding the benign nature of these changes. For example, in **telogen effluvium** (see Chapter 25) the hair will re-grow a few months post-partum. Some changes may persist and may later require treatment to improve the cosmetic appearance. For example, **spider naevi** (Figure 28.1) may be treated with pulsed dye laser and **melasma** (Figure 28.2) with depigmentation treatment (topical hydroquinone, tretinoin and hydrocortisone), sunblock and advice on sun protection.

Skin lesions in pregnancy

The vast majority of skin lesions that change or occur during pregnancy are benign (Figure 28.3) and do not require any active treatment. The differential diagnosis of a rapidly growing lesion during pregnancy is either a pyogenic granuloma or a malignant melanoma, although these are not specifically 'pregnancy-related'.

Pyogenic granulomas (Figure 28.4) commonly occur on fingers, but can develop at any body site. Usually, there is a history of a preceding injury followed by the development of a nodular lesion that bleeds on contact. Pyogenic granulomas are treated by curettage of the lesion followed by cautery of the base of the lesion.

Malignant melanoma (Figure 28.5), although rare, is one of the most common malignancies presenting during pregnancy and may metastasise to the placenta and fetus. A melanoma may arise from a pre-existing naevus or develop *de novo* at any body site. Clinically suspicious lesions should be completely excised promptly for a histological diagnosis (for details on melanoma see Chapter 35).

Pregnancy-related dermatoses

Differentiating between pregnancy-related dermatoses is important because of their effect on the outcome of the pregnancy (Table 28.2).

Polymorphic eruption of pregnancy

This develops in the third trimester or in the immediate post-partum period with extremely itchy urticated papules and plaques. The rash may be widespread or confined to the abdominal wall with characteristic peri-umbilical sparing (Figure 28.6).

Diagnosis is made clinically, it has a benign course and therefore does not require further investigation.

Treatment is aimed at symptomatic relief and consists of topical anti-pruritic treatment (e.g. 1% menthol in aqueous cream), topical corticosteroids and sedative oral anti-histamines (e.g. chlorphenamine).

Pemphigoid gestationis

Pemphigoid gestationis usually develops in the second or third trimester with a widespread, extremely itchy blistering rash. It is thought to occur due to presence of tissue of paternal genetic origin (fetus, hydatidiform mole, choriocarcinoma) and changes in maternal oestrogen and progesterone levels. May recur in subsequent pregnancies with the same partner.

Maternal autoantibodies against the bullous pemphigoid antigen BP180 in the skin basement membrane result in blistering. These autoantibodies may also target the placental basement membrane resulting in placental insufficiency and a 'small for dates' fetus.

Diagnosis is confirmed by skin biopsies for routine histology and direct immunofluorescence (see Chapter 17).

Management: topical anti-pruritic treatment (e.g. 1% menthol in aqueous cream), oral anti-histamine (e.g. chlorphenamine), topical and systemic steroids (oral prednisolone).

Intra-hepatic cholestasis of pregnancy

This can develop during any trimester, commonly the third trimester. Patients present with severe generalised itching and jaundice. Due to the potential adverse effects on the fetus (fetal distress, prematurity, stillbirth), the mother requires close monitoring with measurement of serum bile salts and bilirubin.

Treatment: topical anti-pruritic treatment (e.g. 1% menthol in aqueous cream), oral ursodeoxycholic acid or cholestyramine, or narrowband ultraviolet B (UVB) phototherapy (see Chapter 39).

Effect of pregnancy on pre-existing skin diseases

The effect of pregnancy on pre-existing skin diseases is variable. Psoriasis and acne generally improve, whereas atopic eczema worsens. However, psoriasis and acne may worsen post-partum.

Management of skin diseases during pregnancy

Consideration of the potential risk to the fetus is required when managing any form of skin disease in pregnancy. Bland emollients can be used liberally to moisturise any dry skin condition and provide symptomatic relief from itching. Topical corticosteroids are safe when used sparingly, under medical supervision, for treatment of certain skin diseases during pregnancy (e.g. severe eczema, pemphigoid gestationis, polymorphic eruption of pregnancy).

Narrowband UVB phototherapy is considered safe for the treatment of severe psoriasis, eczema and pruritus from intra-hepatic cholestasis during pregnancy.

Use of systemic treatment for skin diseases is limited because of the potential risk to the fetus during pregnancy. Systemic steroids (e.g. oral prednisolone) may be used, under close supervision, for severe skin diseases during pregnancy such as severe eczema and pemphigoid gestationis.

Erythromycin is the safest systemic option for the treatment of severe acne during pregnancy.

Key points

- Pemphigoid gestationis and intra-hepatic cholestasis of pregnancy can be associated with adverse fetal outcome.
- Risk–benefit ratio to the mother and fetus should be considered in consultation with the obstetrician when using systemic therapy for skin diseases during pregnancy.

▶ **Warning**

A rapidly growing lesion during pregnancy should be surgically excised for histological examination to exclude malignant melanoma.

Table 29.1 **Skin manifestations in the elderly**

- **Benign skin lesions**
  - seborrhoeic keratoses (see Chapter 33)
  - Campbell de Morgan spots
  - solar keratoses (see Chapter 33)

- **Malignant skin lesions**
  - non-melanoma skin cancer (basal cell carcinoma, squamous cell carcinoma) (see Chapter 34)
  - melanoma (see Chapter 35)
  - cutaneous T-cell lymphoma (see Chapter 36)

- **Skin rashes and other skin manifestations**
  - xerosis
  - stasis eczema
  - seborrhoeic dermatitis (see Chapters 20 and 23)
  - psoriasis (see Chapter 12)
  - drug-induced rashes
  - skin manifestations due to systemic causes
  - bullous skin diseases (bullous pemphigoid) (see Chapter 17)
  - skin infections/infestations (tinea pedis, onychomycosis, scabies) (see Chapters 20 and 21)
  - leg and pressure ulcers (see Chapter 45)

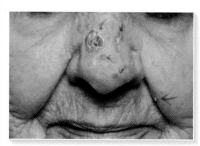

Fig. 29.1
Multiple basal carcinomas on the nose

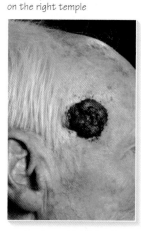

Fig. 29.2
Delayed presentation of a large squamous cell carcinoma on the right temple

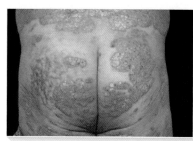

Fig. 29.5
Large plaque psoriasis on the buttocks where the patient had difficulty reaching to apply topical treatment

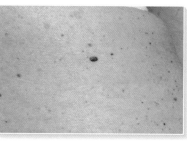

Fig. 29.6
Multiple Campbell de Morgan spots

Fig. 29.3
Chronic venous ulcer with surrounding stasis eczema of the lower leg

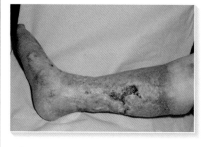

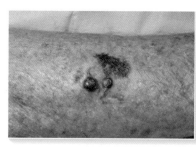

Fig. 29.7
Delayed presentation of a nodular malignant melanoma on the forearm

Fig. 29.4
Eroding nodular basal cell carcinoma of the nose due to delayed presentation

Fig. 29.8 **Xerosis**

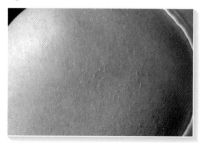

Table 29.2 **Possible causes of xerosis and pruritus in the elderly**

- **Age:** age-related xerosis and pruritus
- **Drug-induced:** diuretics, non-steroidal anti-inflammatory medication
- **Skin diseases/infestations:** eczema, cutaneous T-cell lymphoma, scabies
- **Nutritional deficiencies:** iron deficiency (causing anaemia)
- **Haematological diseases:** lymphoma, myelodysplasia, multiple myeloma
- **Metabolic or endocrine diseases:** renal impairment, liver disease, hypothyroidism, diabetes

Dermatology at a Glance, First Edition. Mahbub M.U. Chowdhury, Ruwani P. Katugampola, and Andrew Y. Finlay.

62 © 2013 John Wiley & Sons, Ltd. Published 2013 by John Wiley & Sons, Ltd.

Skin diseases affecting elderly individuals are summarised in Table 29.1. Elderly patients may present with multiple skin lesions, either benign, malignant or a combination (Figure 29.1).

Attitudes to skin diseases in the elderly

Some elderly patients 'put up' with skin diseases that they consider non-life-threatening. Patients may delay seeking medical attention until the rash or lesion becomes symptomatic (e.g. bleeding basal cell carcinoma or squamous cell carcinoma) (Figure 29.2).

Co-morbidities impacting on skin disease in the elderly

Co-morbidities may be the primary cause, contribute to the skin disease or impact on its management (e.g. impaired mobility due to arthritis may result in stasis eczema or chronic venous leg ulceration) (Figure 29.3).

Memory or visual impairment can also delay presentation until the rash or tumour is more extensive or advanced (Figure 29.4).

Elderly individuals are often on multiple systemic medications, some of which may cause skin diseases (e.g. peri-anal ulceration due to nicorandil). Potential interactions with other medications and exacerbation of other co-morbidities should be borne in mind when starting elderly individuals on systemic treatment for their skin disease (e.g. worsening diabetes with the use of oral steroids).

Factors to consider when managing elderly people with skin diseases

Practicalities of applying topical treatment: elderly patients living alone or those with co-morbidities such as arthritis or poor vision may not be able to apply topical treatments to difficult to reach and/or see body sites (e.g. back) (Figure 29.5). Family members or carers may need to be involved and educated about the topical treatment.

Skin diseases such as eczema or psoriasis require several topical treatments: moisturisers to be applied frequently and all over the skin, and an 'active' treatment such as a topical corticosteroid or vitamin D analogue to be applied for a limited period only to affected skin. A clear written treatment plan to include the name, application site, frequency and duration of specific treatments is helpful. Try to keep it simple.

Those living alone or unable to comply with treatment may benefit from dermatology day care or inpatient treatment.

Benign skin lesions

Common benign skin lesions including those seen in the elderly are described in Chapter 33.

Campbell de Morgan spots

This is one of the most common benign skin lesions occurring in the elderly consisting of dilated capillaries (Figure 29.6). Multiple lesions develop on any body site, often the trunk. They appear as small red (hence the term cherry angiomas) non-blanching macules or papules. Lesions are usually asymptomatic and therefore treatment is not required. Larger lesions, which may be prone to repeated trauma and bleeding, can be treated with electrocautery.

Malignant skin lesions

These are discussed in Chapters 34–36. Malignant lesions in the elderly may be larger and more advanced because of delay in presentation (Figure 29.7).

Xerosis and pruritus

Xerosis (dry skin) (Figure 29.8) and pruritus are common with many possible underlying causes (Table 29.2).

Management of xerosis and pruritus includes a detailed clinical history, with particular attention to the drug history.

In addition to examination for underlying skin diseases or infestation (e.g. scabies), the patient should have a full physical examination, including palpation for lymphadenopathy and hepato-splenomegaly (lymphoma, myelodysplasia). Blood investigations should include a full blood count, renal and liver function, thyroid function, glucose, ferritin, serum immunoglobulins and electrophoresis.

Further investigations include a blood film, urine Bence-Jones proteins, creatinine clearance, ultrasound scan of the liver, spleen and kidneys, and biopsy of skin, lymph node or bone marrow.

In addition to treating the underlying cause, symptomatic treatment for xerosis and pruritus includes topical emollients (especially with urea or lactic acid base), topical anti-pruritic agents (e.g. 1% menthol in aqueous cream), avoidance of soap and use of soap substitutes, bath emollients (caution elderly patients about the risk of slipping in the bath) and oral anti-histamines.

Bullous pemphigoid

Bullous pemphioid is an autoimmune bullous skin disease that mainly affects elderly individuals and is described in Chapter 17.

Pre-bullous pemphigoid can present as intense pruritus in an elderly patient prior to the development of the tense blisters.

Localised disease can be managed with super-potent topical corticosteroids such as clobetasol propionate. Widespread disease requires a tapering dose of systemic steroids (e.g. prednisolone initiating at 40 mg/day) with an immunosuppressant such as mycophenolate mofetil or azathioprine.

Key points

- Elderly individuals may present with advanced skin malignancies because of delayed presentation.
- Underlying malignancy needs to be excluded in patients presenting with xerosis and pruritus.
- Elderly patients on prolonged systemic steroid treatment should be monitored for hypertension and diabetes, and given prophylaxis for osteoporosis and gastritis.

Table 30.1 **Indications for patch testing**

- Atopic dermatitis
- Hand dermatitis
- Other dermatoses e.g. discoid, stasis, seborrhoeic
- Specific site dermatitis e.g. eyelids, foot, perineal
- Occupational dermatitis

Fig. 30.1 **Mechanisms of type I and type IV allergy**

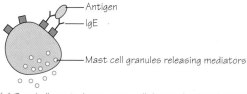

- Antigen
- IgE
- Mast cell granules releasing mediators

(a) Type I allergy is due to mast cell degranulation releasing mediators such as histamine

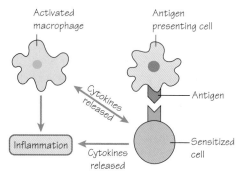

Activated macrophage

Antigen presenting cell

Cytokines released

Antigen

Inflammation

Cytokines released

Sensitized cell

(b) Type IV allergy requires antigen-presenting cells to bind the antigen and to present this to T-cells inducing allergen-specific T-cells. Further contact with the antigen will release cytokines to activate macrophages, leading to inflammation and further proliferation of allergen-specific memory T-cells

Table 30.2 **Common examples of allergens tested**

Potassium dichromate	Leather, cement
4-Phenylenediamine base	Hair dye
Thiuram mix	Rubber accelerator
Nickel	Metal, jewellery
Colophony	Pine resin, adhesives, printing ink
Paraben mix	Preservatives in creams
Wool alcohols	Ointment base in creams
Epoxy resin	Resin in adhesives
Balsam of Peru	Perfumes & flavouring agent
Mercaptobenzothiazole	Rubber chemical
Formaldehyde	Disinfectant, cosmetic preservative
Fragrance mix	Perfumes
Sesquiterpene lactone mix	Plants e.g. chrysanthemum
Tixocortol-21-pivalate	Topical steroids (hydrocortisone)

Fig. 30.2 **Overlap of dermatitis types**

Endogenous dermatitis

Allergic contact dermatitis

Irritant contact dermatitis

Allergic contact dermatitis, irritant contact dermatitis and endogenous dermatitis often occur together

Fig. 30.3 **Hand eczema**

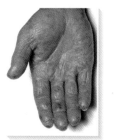

Fig. 30.4
Irritant contact dermatitis
– note scaling in webspaces

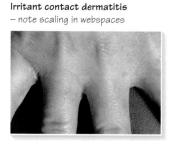

Fig. 30.5
Severe pompholyx with vesicles

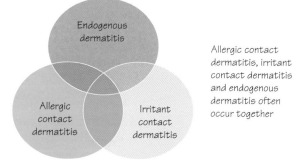

Fig. 30.6 **Patches ready to apply**

Fig. 30.7
Patches applied to back

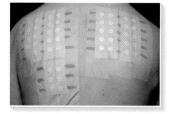

Fig. 30.8
Nickel allergy with vesicles

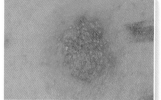

Fig. 30.9
Strong hair dye allergy with blisters

Fig. 30.10
Multiple positive skin prick test reactions

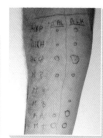

Dermatology at a Glance, First Edition. Mahbub M.U. Chowdhury, Ruwani P. Katugampola, and Andrew Y. Finlay.

64 © 2013 John Wiley & Sons, Ltd. Published 2013 by John Wiley & Sons, Ltd.

Contact dermatitis can be irritant or allergic and occurs when a substance or chemical comes into contact with the skin.

- 5% of all dermatology presentations are due to contact dermatitis.
- 50% of occupational disease may be due to dermatitis.

Hairdressers, beauticians, florists, machine operators, printers and metalworkers are more prone to contact dermatitis.

Hand eczema is very common and up to 25% of women will have this at some time during their life (Figure 30.3).

Irritant contact dermatitis

Irritant contact dermatitis (ICD) is the result of localised toxic effects of an irritant on the skin.

ICD accounts for approximately 80% of all contact dermatitis, while allergic contact dermatitis (ACD) accounts for only 20%. This is often in contrast to the patient's suspicions as they frequently link skin eruptions with an allergy.

Patients with ICD present with redness, scaling and fissures on the skin, especially the dorsal and palmar surfaces of the hands, but it may occur mainly in the finger web spaces (Figure 30.4). The definitive diagnosis of ICD needs confirmation by exclusion of ACD with patch testing.

Allergic contact dermatitis

ACD is a type IV or delayed (T-lymphocyte mediated) hypersensitivity reaction. Type IV allergy requires antigen presenting cells (APC) in the epidermis (e.g. dendritic Langerhans cells) to bind the antigen to major histocompatibility complex (MHC) Class II proteins. APC travel to the draining lymph nodes via lymphatics and activate T cells by presenting this complex. These T cells then release cytokines (e.g. IL-2) to activate macrophages leading to proliferation of allergen-specific memory T cells (sensitization) (Figure 30.1b). On further encountering the same antigen (allergen) these T cells will migrate to the site of skin contact to release further cytokines and cause inflammation (elicitation).

ACD occurs much less frequently than ICD but is of great importance as it can frequently force a worker to change jobs as protective measures often fail to work. When chronic, ICD and ACD can look quite similar clinically; however, vesicles are more common in ACD. Vesicles can also occur in endogenous pompholyx eczema, especially on the sides of fingers (Figure 30.5). ACD and ICD can be difficult to differentiate and may co-exist.

Treatment of ACD consists of identifying the relevant allergen, treating the current problem with topical or systemic treatment (e.g. oral prednisolone) and educating the patient to avoid contact with the allergen.

Patch testing

Patch testing is a specialized technique where allergens are applied to the patient's back to detect delayed hypersensitivity (Tables 30.1 and 30.2).

The test involves three visits in 1 week with patches applied on Day 0 (Monday), patches removed and first reading on Day 2 (Wednesday) and final reading on Day 4 (Friday).

The allergens (chemicals) tested are usually placed in Finn chambers. These 8-mm aluminium pots are placed on an adhesive tape in strips of 10 (Figure 30.6).

A standard patch test series was put together in the 1980s in order to standardize patch testing and is regularly updated. This series aims to test an individual patient to the most common allergens (around 40 allergens) encountered in the environment. Additional series (e.g. hairdresser or cosmetic series) can be added if the investigator feels this is necessary. Up to 60–80 allergens can be tested on the backs of most adults (Figure 30.7).

Reactions are graded by intensity of papules, vesicles and blisters under the applied patch test allergen. Stronger reactions indicate the specific allergen is more likely to be relevant to the patient's current skin problem. Common examples are nickel and hair dye allergy (Figures 30.8 and 30.9).

Prick testing

Type 1 allergy is caused by mast cell degranulation releasing mediators such as histamine (Figure 30.1a). Prick testing is primarily used to detect allergens causing type 1 (IgE mediated) or acute hypersensitivity reactions. Anti-histamines should be stopped 2–4 days prior to the test.

In this test a small needle is used to gently prick the skin through a drop of fluid containing a known allergen. This allows a small quantity of allergen into the dermis (Figure 30.10).

A positive control (histamine) and negative control (saline) are used to compare skin reactivity. Reactions (at 15 minutes) larger (2–3 mm greater in diameter) than the saline reaction or at least 50% of the histamine reaction diameter are taken as positive.

Solutions containing antigens are available commercially for many allergens including latex, house dust mite, animal fur, trees, grasses and various food products.

Management and prognosis of contact dermatitis

- Skin protection with suitable gloves, regular emollients and hand care is essential.
- Avoidance of irritants and allergens causing the dermatitis.
- Allergen avoidance needs to be strict and it can take up to 6 weeks to see any benefit in the skin.
- If any improvement occurs then continued avoidance is essential and indicates a good prognosis.

Key points

- ICD is more common than ACD.
- Always think of contact allergy in non-resolving dermatitis.
- Overlap of ICD, ACD and endogenous eczema is common.

► Warning

Prick test with care (resuscitation facilities) if the patient has a history of anaphylaxis.

31 The working hands

Table 31.1 **Types of Hand Eczema and other differentials**

- **Psoriasis:** Sharp, well demarcated edges of silvery scaly patches or plaques, symmetrical and little itching, worse with friction. Other clues include scaly scalp, nail pitting, extensor surface of elbows and knees affected (see Fig. 31.1)
- **Hyperkeratotic hand eczema:** Increased itching compared to psoriasis. Can be difficult to distinguish as can have sharp margins with fissures also (Fig. 31.2)
- **Tinea manuum:** May be unilateral on palms. Can affect manual workers e.g. with wet work. Scaly, inflamed leading edge (with or without tinea pedis) (Fig. 31.3)
- **Pompholyx:** Vesicles can be extremely itchy on lateral sides of fingers and palms, healing with scaling (see Fig. 31.4)
- **Irritant contact dermatitis:** Scaling in web spaces and dorsum of hands with no vesicles (see Fig. 31.5)
- **Allergic contact dermatitis:** Vesicles can be present (not diagnostic) (see Fig. 31.6)
- **Atopic hand eczema:** Atopy including asthma and hayfever. Previous history in childhood of atopic eczema affecting flexures. Apron pattern of eczema at the base of the fingers (see Fig. 31.7)

Table 31.2 **Occupations predisposed to Hand Irritation** (and causes)

- **Hairdressers** (due to hand washing, shampoos) (see Fig. 31.5)
- **Nurses** (hand washing, alcohol gels)
- **Mechanics** (oils, detergents)
- **Chefs** (raw vegetables, fish)
- **Butchers** (hand washing, meats)

Occupations predisposed to Allergy (and causes)

- **Construction workers** (chromium in cement)
- **Hairdressers** (hair dyes, nickel)
- **Florists** (plants e.g. chrysanthemums) (see Fig. 31.6)
- **Aromatherapists** (perfumes, essential oils)
- **Rubber workers** (natural latex, preservatives in processing)
- **Metal workers** (nickel, cobalt, chromium)

Table 31.3
Treatment for Hand Eczema

- **Topical corticosteroids** (with occlusion)
- **Oral corticosteroids**
- **Hand PUVA**
- **Immunosuppressants** e.g. azathioprine, ciclosporin, methotrexate
- **Retinoids** e.g. alitretinoin

Fig. 31.7
Apron pattern in endogenous eczema
i.e. like an 'apron on 2 legs'

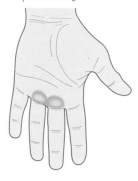

Fig. 31.1a/b
Thickened scaly psoriasis plaques on palms

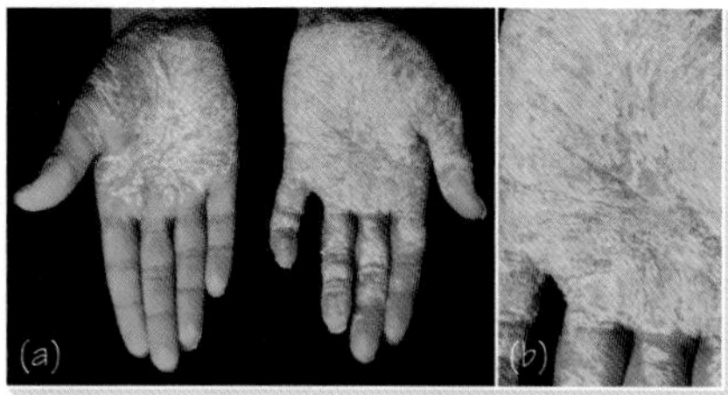

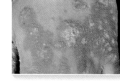

Fig. 31.1f
Typical silvery scaling on dorsum hand

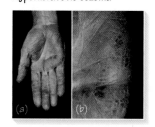

Fig. 31.2a/b
Hyperkeratotic eczema

Fig. 31.2c
Note visible peeling on palm

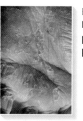

Fig. 31.1c/d **Note painful fissures on both hands**

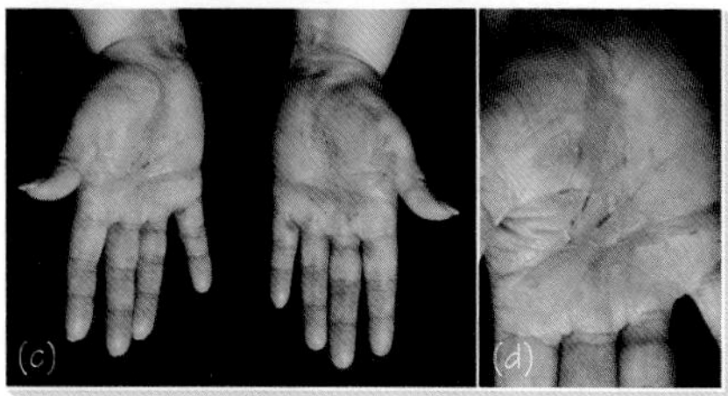

Fig. 31.1g/h
Severe pustulosis with brown macules

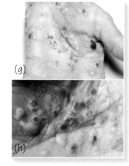

Fig. 31.3a/b
Tinea manuum in manual worker

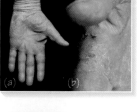

Fig. 31.4
Note itchy vesicles on palm

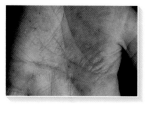

Fig. 31.1e
Hyperkeratotic psoriasis at friction sites

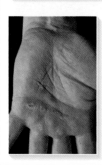

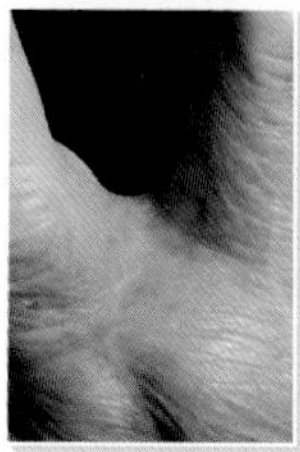

Fig. 31.5
Irritant dermatitis in hairdresser

Fig. 31.6
Dominant hand of florist with chrysan-themum allergy

Dermatology at a Glance, First Edition. Mahbub M.U. Chowdhury, Ruwani P. Katugampola, and Andrew Y. Finlay.

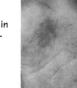

Problems with the skin on the hands are very common, accounting for 90% of all occupational skin diseases. Hand dermatitis has a prevalence of 5–10% in the population with an incidence of around 5% per year. Psoriasis, tinea infections and atopic eczema including pompholyx mainly affect the hands (Table 31.1). Endogenous dermatitis, allergic contact dermatitis and irritant contact dermatitis need to be differentiated by detailed history, examination and investigations such as patch testing (see Chapter 30).

Hand eczema

Patients with chronic hand eczema tend to have prolonged sick leave, increased health costs and decreased quality of life. Each year 60% of people with hand eczema visit their GP and up to 20% visit a specialist. Twenty-five per cent of chronic hand eczema is caused by allergic contact dermatitis.

Poor prognosis for hand eczema is associated with atopy (especially respiratory), contact allergy, older age, increased severity and longer duration (>1 year) of eczema. Other factors are patient exposure to wet work, increased frequency of hand washing and wearing gloves for long periods of time (>4–6 hours/day).

Thirty per cent of nurses develop hand eczema. Senior nurses with atopy, multiple hand washes during the day and wearing gloves for prolonged periods of time are particularly at risk. This is mainly a result of irritant contact dermatitis; however, allergic contact dermatitis needs to be excluded with patch testing.

Apprentice hairdressers have a high risk of hand eczema because of excess wet work and exposure to irritant and potentially allergenic chemicals (e.g. nickel, hair dyes). Up to 35% develop hand eczema within 2 years. Up to 30% of people in occupations at high risk of hand eczema (e.g. food industry, builders, hairdressers) may need to change their occupation, leading to a better prognosis medically.

Intervention with correct diagnosis and early treatment within 1 year of presentation leads to a better prognosis.

Prevention of hand eczema

The focus of any prevention should be at early stages for those at risk.

Primary and secondary prevention involves education of skin care for professions with increased risk. Important factors include elimination of relevant contact factors such as irritants and potential allergens.

Maintenance of the skin barrier function is essential with skin care education and skin protection. Skin protection includes personal protection equipment such as gloves and gauntlets (long gloves with forearm protection). Simple measures, such as reducing the amount of hand washing, are very effective.

Occupational hand eczema caused by conditions such as type 1 natural rubber latex allergy in health care workers can be prevented by using low allergenic powder-free latex gloves. Hand eczema can be controlled with avoidance of latex gloves and using alternatives such as nitrile or vinyl gloves. Prognosis in health care workers with this diagnosis can be very favourable with these simple measures.

Certain occupations are pre-disposed to problems with 'working hands' with regards to irritation and allergic contact dermatitis (Table 31.2). Specific treatment for other hand diseases is determined by the diagnosis (e.g. psoriasis or tinea manuum).

Treatment (Table 31.3)

Hand protection needs to be undertaken and regular emollients and soap substitutes used with avoidance of irritants. Topical or oral corticosteroids can be used for other causes of hand eczema including pompholyx.

Topical steroids may need to be used at very high potency for a short period of time (e.g. clobetasol propionate [Dermovate®] for 6 weeks). Topical steroids can be used under occlusion to get adequate absorption using cling film or cotton gloves. Oral steroids can be used but there is a risk of rebound flare once they are stopped.

Topical PUVA therapy can be used for the hands for a period of 8–10 weeks (20–30 treatments).

Any infection confirmed with skin swabs should be treated with systemic and topical antibiotics. Systemic therapies such as alitretinoin (oral retinoid) are recommended by the National Institute for Clinical Excellence (NICE) to be used after potent topical steroids (e.g. clobetasol propionate [Dermovate®]) if Dermatology Life Quality Index is >15 and the physician's assessment is of severe hand eczema.

Immunosuppressants used include azathioprine, ciclosporin and methotrexate. These can be effective in selected patients even though they are not licensed for use in hand eczema.

Key points

- Hand eczema accounts for 90% of all occupational skin disease patients.
- Hand eczema has a poorer prognosis in atopic individuals especially if severe with a long history.
- Contact allergy to allergens such as chrome may lead to persistent hand eczema even after avoidance of the allergen.
- Hand psoriasis can look similar to hyperkeratotic hand eczema.
- Consider all differentials for work-related hand skin disease and review the diagnosis if there is no improvement.

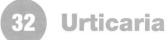

Table 32.1 Causes of urticaria

- **Drugs:** aspirin, non-steroidal anti-inflammatory drugs (NSAIDs), angiotensin converting enzyme inhibitors, omeprazole and simvastatin
- **Antibiotics:** penicillins, cephalosporins and tetracyclines
- **Foods:** fish, milk, potatoes, carrots, spices, bananas, shellfish and hazelnuts
- **Food additives:** tartrazine and azo dyes including sunset yellow, benzoates, sulphites
- **Infections:** viral and bacterial such as dental sepsis, sinusitis, gall bladder and urinary tract

Table 32.2 Enquiries for history taking in urticaria

- **Comprehensive history required:** onset, disease course, duration of individual wheals, presence of purpura or angio-oedema
- **Systemic symptoms:** malaise, headache, abdominal pain, wheezing and syncope
- **Precipitating factors:** heat, cold, pressure, friction, sunlight, latex
- **Drug history:** aspirin, NSAIDs, antibiotics, over the counter medication
- **Other history:** association with any recent infection, foods, family history of angio-oedema

Table 32.3 Investigations in urticaria

- Exclude associated conditions including full blood count, ESR, thyroid function (5% of chronic urticaria have abnormal thyroid function)
- Skin biopsy if urticarial vasculitis suspected
- Food diary
- Chart of frequency and severity on scale 0–10 (to monitor any change)

If angio-oedema prominent:

- C1 esterase inhibitor level and complement C2, C4 (may be reduced in hereditary angio-oedema)
- Complement C3, C4 (may be reduced in urticarial vasculitis)

Table 32.4 Drug treatments

- **Urticaria**
  - classic H1 antihistamines: chlorphenamine, hydroxyzine
  - second generation H1 antihistamines: cetirizine, loratidine, fexofenadine
  - tricyclic antidepressant: doxepin
  - H2 antagonists: ranitidine, cimetidine
  - corticosteroids
- **Non-hereditary angio-oedema**
  - epinephrine (EpiPen®)
  - ciclosporin
  - intravenous immunoglobulins
- **Hereditary angio-oedema**
  - androgens: danazol and stanozolol
  - epsilon (aminocaproic acid)
  - tranexamic acid
  - fresh frozen plasma

Table 32.5 Types of physical urticaria

- Delayed pressure
- Vibration
- Exercise, heat, cold
- Sun exposure
- Aquagenic urticaria
- Contact urticaria

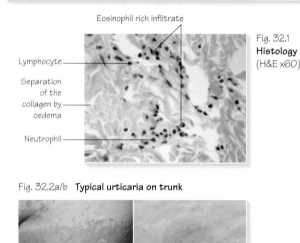

Fig. 32.1 **Histology (H&E x60)**

Eosinophil rich infiltrate · Lymphocyte · Separation of the collagen by oedema · Neutrophil

Fig. 32.2a/b **Typical urticaria on trunk**

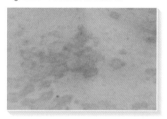

Fig. 32.3 **Annular urticaria**

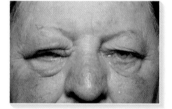

Fig. 32.5 **Angio-oedema of eyelids**

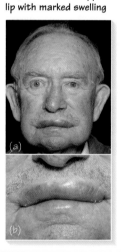

Fig. 32.4a/b **Angio-oedema of upper lip with marked swelling**

Urticaria is a common condition which can present to many different physicians including dermatologists, immunologists and GPs.

Urticaria is known as 'nettle rash', itchy hives or wheals. It is a temporary eruption of erythema and oedema with swelling of the dermis and is usually itchy. Urticaria and angio-oedema (deeper dermal and subcutaneous swellings) may occur together.

Classification

Urticaria can be classified as ordinary urticaria consisting of acute or chronic urticaria. Urticaria is defined as chronic if lasting >6 weeks. A cause is less likely to be found than for acute urticaria. Other types include physical and cholinergic, contact urticaria and immune complex urticaria such as urticarial vasculitis.

Histology and pathophysiology

Histology of ordinary urticaria wheals shows oedema and perivascular mixed cellular (eosinophils, lymphocytes, neutrophils) dermal infiltrate with vascular and lymphatic dilatation (Figure 32.1). Electron microscopy may show dermal mast cell degranulation.

Pathophysiology of urticaria includes increased capillary and venous permeability. Cutaneous mast cell activation releases mediators including histamine leading to activation of H1 receptors which induces itching, erythema and whealing.

Other histamine releasing factors involved include tryptase and neuropeptides (substance P). Plasma mediators (bradykinin) and complement may play a part in angio-oedema with complement activation leading to immune complex urticaria and urticarial vasculitis.

Clinical features

Urticaria presents as itchy erythematous macules and wheals with pink swollen raised areas with a surrounding flare (Figure 32.2). The sites affected are variable and can include the palms and soles. The number, shape and size of the lesions vary with bizarre shapes including annular patterns (Figure 32.3). In ordinary urticaria the wheals resolve within 24 hours and may last only a few hours. They leave no skin change.

Fifty per cent of patients with urticaria may have angio-oedema of the face, lips (Figure 32.4), eyelids (Figure 32.5), hands and genitalia (see Chapter 16). Mucosal swellings can occur inside the mouth (e.g. tongue, pharynx and larynx). Occasionally, systemic symptoms associated with urticaria include vomiting, general malaise, headache and abdominal pain with syncopy and in severe forms anaphylaxis.

In urticarial vasculitis, lesions last >24 hours and can leave bruises. Skin biopsy is essential to confirm this diagnosis.

Causes (Table 32.1)

Acute urticaria has no identifiable cause in 30% of patients. Acute allergic urticaria may be caused by an IgE-mediated mast cell degranulation. The most common causes are drugs, foods and, rarely, food additives.

Chronic urticaria has wheals that last for >6 weeks and 40% may have physical urticaria (e.g. delayed pressure urticaria). Most are idiopathic as only 10–20% have an identifiable cause.

Potential exacerbating factors of urticaria include drugs such as aspirin or non-steroidal anti-inflammatory drugs (NSAIDs) and viral or bacterial infections but treatment of these infections does not always clear the chronic urticaria.

Prognosis

Acute urticaria attacks may last for a few hours a day and then fade. Chronic cases, particularly if idiopathic, may last for weeks, months or even years. Fifty per cent of patients with urticaria can be clear within 6–12 months.

Management

Detailed history and some investigations may be necessary (Tables 32.2 and 32.3).

Reassurance regarding the diagnosis is needed. Reducing stress and alcohol, avoidance of aspirin and salicylates, NSAIDs and opiates are helpful.

Diets may need to exclude food additives, colourings or preservatives if these substances are detected as causative agents.

Drug management (Table 32.4)

As urticaria is histamine mediated, H1 receptor blockers (antihistamines) can reduce itch, whealing and erythema. Classic antihistamines such as chlorphenamine have side effects of sedation and anti-cholinergic properties but are useful for night-time sedation and to reduce itching. Second generation H1 anti-histamines are the treatment of choice with low levels of sedation and minimal anti-cholinergic side effects. Regular anti-histamines may need to be used for long periods to have satisfactory control of the urticaria.

Corticosteroids are effective in patients with severe urticaria and short courses of oral steroids are often prescribed for acute exacerbations. However, prolonged use must be avoided because of the risk of side effects and also instability of the urticaria once the prednisolone is stopped. This makes further control of the urticaria extremely difficult.

Non-hereditary angio-oedema with respiratory involvement may require epinephrine (adrenaline) which causes rapid vasoconstriction. Treatment may need to be repeated if there is no improvement within 10–20 minutes and self-administration of epinephrine (EpiPen®) may be required in the future (see Chapter 16).

Physical and cholinergic urticarias

This is a distinct group of patients with a physical cause for the whealing (Table 32.5). Cholinergic urticaria can be linked with heat and sweating. Physical urticaria causes approximately 20% of urticaria with dermographism which is the triple response arising from firm stroking of the skin. This involves local erythema with capillary vasodilatation followed by oedema and surrounding flare. This is normal in 5% of people and if exaggerated is called dermographism. Clinically, this may present as whealing and itching at sites of trauma and friction with clothing. These types are less common and management requires avoidance of the cause and anti-histamines.

Hereditary angio-oedema

This is very rare (5% of angio-oedema) and occurs without urticaria. A family history is usually present (autosomal dominant trait on chromosome 11). The condition starts in childhood but can be delayed into late adult life. Recurrent swellings of the skin and mucous membranes occur with nausea, vomiting, abdominal colic and urinary symptoms. Swelling of the pharynx, larynx and bronchial tree can occur leading to death. Results of therapy with conventional anti-histamines are poor. Androgens may be effective but replacement therapy with fresh frozen plasma for short-term prophylaxis may be needed (Table 32.4).

Key points

- Acute urticaria usually lasts <6 weeks.
- Chronic urticaria can be long lasting (years) with no cause found in 80% of patients.
- Management of urticaria can be difficult requiring combination of anti-histamines.

► Warning

Corticosteroid therapy makes further control of urticaria extremely difficult.

Table 33.1

Classification of benign lesions based on derivation

- **Epidermis:** Seborrhoeic wart, solar keratosis, Bowen's disease
- **Melanocytes:** Freckle, lentigo, melanocytic naevus
- **Hair follicles:** Epidermoid cyst
- **Fibroblasts:** Dermatofibroma

Fig. 33.1
Junctional naevus
– flat and dark

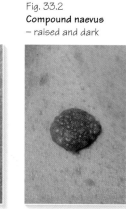

Fig. 33.2
Compound naevus
– raised and dark

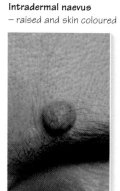

Fig. 33.3
Intradermal naevus
– raised and skin coloured

Fig. 33.4 **Freckles**

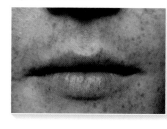

Fig. 33.6
Lentigo maligna
– irregular pigmented area. Needs skin biopsy

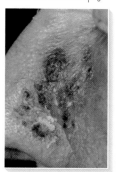

Fig. 33.5
Solar lentigo – regular shaped pigmented macule

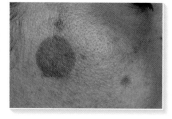

Fig. 33.7
Seborrhoeic wart

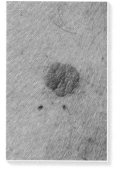

Fig. 33.8
Pigmented seborrhoeic wart

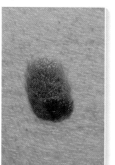

Fig. 33.9a
Cyst with punctum

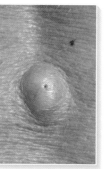

Fig. 33.9b
Large pilar cyst on scalp

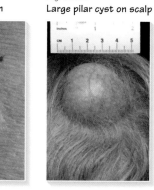

Fig. 33.10
Dermatofibroma
– can be pigmented

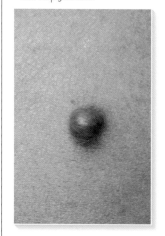

Fig. 33.11a/b
Skin tags

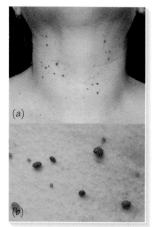

Fig. 33.12a
Cutaneous horn on cheek

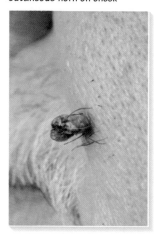

Fig. 33.12b
Cutaneous horn on ear

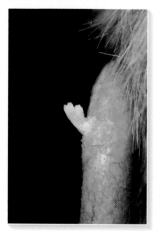

Dermatology at a Glance, First Edition. Mahbub M.U. Chowdhury, Ruwani P. Katugampola, and Andrew Y. Finlay.

70 © 2013 John Wiley & Sons, Ltd. Published 2013 by John Wiley & Sons, Ltd.

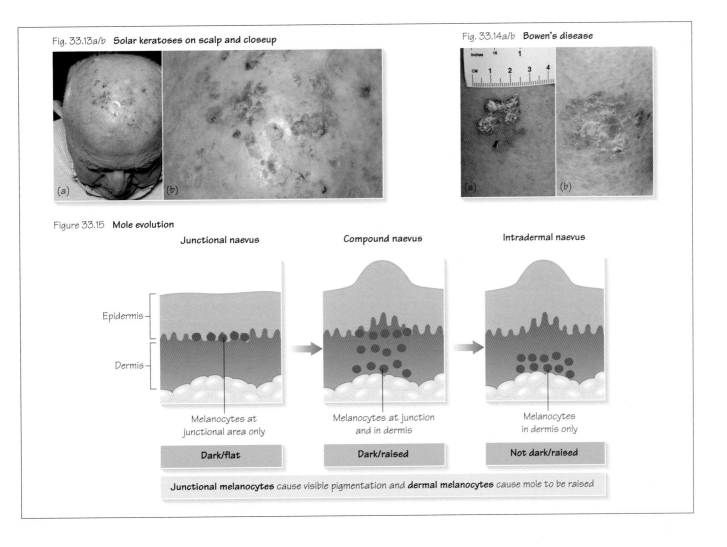

Fig. 33.13a/b Solar keratoses on scalp and closeup

(a) (b)

Fig. 33.14a/b Bowen's disease

(a) (b)

Figure 33.15 Mole evolution

Junctional naevus   Compound naevus   Intradermal naevus

Epidermis

Dermis

Melanocytes at
junctional area only

Melanocytes at junction
and in dermis

Melanocytes
in dermis only

Dark/flat   Dark/raised   Not dark/raised

Junctional melanocytes cause visible pigmentation and dermal melanocytes cause mole to be raised

Benign skin lesions are very common and constitute a large number of skin consultations in general practice. It is important to be able to make a confident correct clinical diagnosis to reassure the patient or to suggest further appropriate management which may include surgical removal.

It is essential that the patient understands the lesion is likely to be benign prior to embarking on a procedure that may lead to a less than ideal cosmetic appearance, hence leading to patient dissatisfaction.

When considering these lesions it is important to think about their derivation (Table 33.1).

Benign melanocytic naevi

These consist of three main types: junctional, compound and intra-dermal melanocytic naevi. These are all benign and are called moles. These are common and appear in childhood and puberty and can become smaller in later life. It is not unusual to see up to 30 naevi in sun exposed areas. However, those with fair skin, a family history of moles and increased sun exposure are likely to have larger numbers (>40).

A melanocytic naevus can change through the three stages from a junctional naevus (usually flat and dark) to a compound naevus (raised and usually dark) to an intradermal naevus (usually flesh coloured) (Figures 33.1–33.3 and 33.15).

• As a **junctional naevus** is flat and brown, a new mole may be difficult to differentiate from malignant melanoma and hence may need to be excised for histology (Figure 33.1). If confident that it is a mole, it can be left alone or excised with a narrow 2 mm margin.

• A **compound melanocytic naevus** is raised, pigmented and can be hairy. Again, if the diagnosis is confident, it can be left alone (Figure 33.2). A shave excision is better cosmetically than a full ellipse excision for these moles. The patient should be warned regarding the likely cosmetic result of a flat scar and that pigmentation and hairs can regrow within the area.

• An **intradermal naevus** is usually raised and non-pigmented and needs to be differentiated from a basal cell carcinoma (BCC) (Figure 33.3).

Freckles and lentigos

Freckles are common benign lesions that usually occur on sun exposed areas and consist of multiple pigmented macules that darken after sun exposure (Figure 33.4). These start in childhood and do not have an increase in melanocytes but the melanosomes within the melanocytes produce increased melanin in response to sun exposure.

A **lentigo** can also be a small pigmented macule but the pigmentation is the result of an increase in the number of melanocytes in the basal layer and does not darken significantly after sun exposure (Figure 33.5). They are solitary, occur on sun exposed skin and can be termed solar lentigines. Lesions that are larger may need to be excised for diagnosis to exclude a lentigo maligna (Hutchinson's freckle). This is a pre-malignant melanocytic lesion that usually occurs on the face and can transform to a lentigo maligna melanoma (Figure 33.6).

Seborrhoeic keratosis (basal cell papilloma)

Seborrhoeic keratoses (warts) are benign and very common, especially on the trunk of elderly patients. They are multiple superficial crusted lesions with a greasy appearance, with new lesions developing over time. Size can vary from few millimetres up to 3 cm in diameter. The lesions have a 'stuck-on' appearance and seem to be superficially attached to the dermis (Figure 33.7). The crusted surface can fall off but usually recurs and can be of variable dark colours causing confusion with malignant melanoma (Figure 33.8). They are asymptomatic but can be very itchy and become inflamed or irritated after trauma. Follicular plugged areas can be seen with a dermatoscope which can be extremely helpful for diagnosis. They are best managed with reassurance and explanation of the diagnosis. Usually, they do not need to be removed but if symptomatic or disfiguring can be removed with shave excision, curettage and cautery or cryotherapy (see Chapters 8 and 9). Histology should be checked for solitary lesions.

Epidermoid cyst

Cysts are derived from pilar units and often incorrectly called 'sebaceous cysts'. An epidermoid cyst has an epidermal wall surrounding a core of keratin. These cysts are common in young to middle-aged adults and are usually asymptomatic. If they become inflamed and infected then excision may be warranted as they particularly occur on the head, neck and upper trunk. The lesion is within the dermis with overlying normal epidermis and a punctum (opening on the skin surface) (Figure 33.9a). The pilar type cyst is more common on the scalp (Figure 33.9b) and can be genetically inherited. Contents of cysts are foul smelling and have a cheesy appearance.

Dermatofibroma (histiocytoma)

This consists of a proliferation of fibroblasts in the dermis. This is thought to be often caused by an insect bite which is usually not noticed in most patients. They are common on the lower limbs of women, presenting as a firm hard nodule which can be itchy (Figure 33.10). Some can be pigmented and cause confusion with benign moles. A useful sign for diagnosis is dimpling on the surface when pressure is exerted laterally on both sides of the dermatofibroma. If the diagnosis is clear then excision should not be undertaken for cosmetic reasons as healing can be poor, particularly on the lower limbs. If excised, ellipse excision is the best option.

Skin tag (fibro-epithelial polyp)

Skin tags are extremely common and present as multiple small pedunculated fleshy skin-coloured lesions, increasing in size and number with age and occurring in the axillae, groins and neck (Figure 33.11). Snip excision with cautery is the best treatment if requested.

Solar keratoses (actinic keratoses)

These are common pre-malignant lesions occurring on chronic light exposed skin of fair skinned individuals. The risk of malignant transformation to squamous cell carcinoma (SCC) is extremely small. However, these lesions are treated as they are often multiple. They can be asymptomatic or itch and can present as a cutaneous horn (Figure 33.12). Common sites are the backs of hands, face, scalp and ears and they typically present as multiple pink, rough scaly or crusted lesions (Figure 33.13). Any increase in inflammation or size should be biopsied or excised to exclude SCC. General management of solar keratoses involves sun protection with sunscreen and clothing. Individual lesions are treated with liquid nitrogen cryotherapy, curettage and cautery, topical 5-fluorouracil (Efudix®) or 3% diclofenac gel (Solaraze®).

Bowen's disease (intra-epidermal squamous cell carcinoma)

This is a pre-malignant condition that is less common than solar keratosis and can progress to SCC. Sun exposure (and previously arsenic containing tonics) can lead to Bowen's disease which presents as well-defined persistent inflamed scaly patches on the lower limbs of the elderly (Figure 33.14). Differential diagnoses include superficial BCC, psoriasis, discoid eczema and fungal infections. Surgical excision may be difficult as Bowen's disease occurs commonly on the lower limbs. Other treatments are liquid nitrogen cryotherapy, topical 5-fluorouracil (Efudix®) and imiquimod (Aldara®).

Key points

- Reassure the patient that the lesion is benign if you are 100% certain.
- Warn the patient explicitly regarding possible scar and poor cosmesis with any treatment to remove benign lesions.

▶ Warning

- Do not treat a benign lesion unless the patient is 100% sure he or she wants to proceed.
- Removal of benign moles may leave residual pigment and hair growth.

Table 34.1

High risk factors for non-melanoma skin cancers

- Site: face, lips, ears
- Histology: poor differentiation
- Ill-defined tumour
- Previous incomplete treatment
- Recurrent tumour

Fig. 34.1

Basal cell carcinoma (BCC)
– note typical telangiectasia and shiny appearance

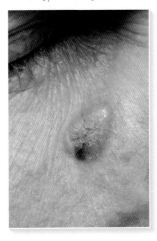

Fig. 34.2

Longstanding BCC with ulceration and pigmentation

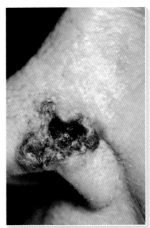

Fig. 34.3a/b

Superficial BCC on left leg
– needs biopsy to confirm diagnosis

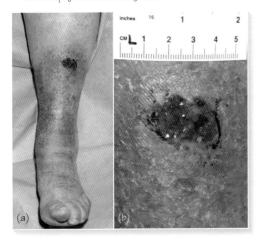

Fig. 34.4a/b

Ill-defined morphoeic BCC on nose

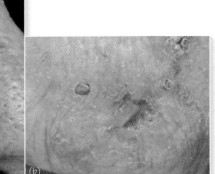

Fig. 34.5 **BCC histology** (H&E x20)

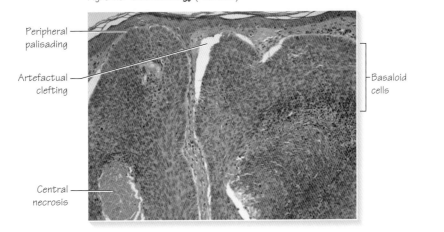

Peripheral palisading

Artefactual clefting

Basaloid cells

Central necrosis

Dermatology at a Glance, First Edition. Mahbub M.U. Chowdhury, Ruwani P. Katugampola, and Andrew Y. Finlay.
© 2013 John Wiley & Sons, Ltd. Published 2013 by John Wiley & Sons, Ltd.

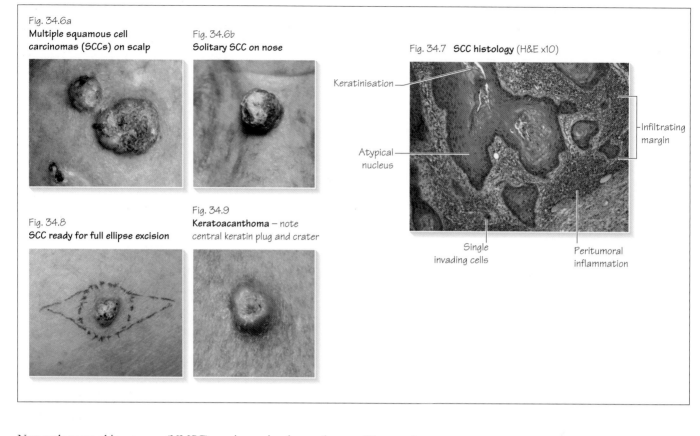

Fig. 34.6a
Multiple squamous cell carcinomas (SCCs) on scalp

Fig. 34.6b
Solitary SCC on nose

Fig. 34.7 SCC histology (H&E x10)

Keratinisation

Atypical nucleus

Infiltrating margin

Single invading cells

Peritumoral inflammation

Fig. 34.8
SCC ready for full ellipse excision

Fig. 34.9
Keratoacanthoma – note central keratin plug and crater

Non-melanoma skin cancers (NMSC) are increasing in number because of the larger elderly population. NMSCs are less likely to metastasise than melanomas.

Basal cell carcinoma ('rodent ulcer')

Basal cell carcinoma (BCC) is also known as a 'rodent ulcer' as the surface can be damaged and ulcerated. BCC is the most common skin and human malignancy and occurs on sun exposed areas of the head and neck in the elderly. With increasing sun exposure BCCs now affect younger adults in their thirties and forties. BCCs grow very slowly but can be locally invasive.

Nodulocystic BCC is the most common type. It usually develops on the face as a pearly skin-coloured cystic papule or nodule with telangiectasia and a rolled edge. It can ulcerate and there may be a history of bleeding or crusting (Figures 34.1 and 34.2). The lesion can be pigmented causing confusion with a melanoma.

Superficial BCC is the second most common type, usually appearing on the trunk as scaly pink to red–brown patches or papules and can have a pearly border (Figure 34.3). The differential diagnoses include Bowen's disease and inflammatory conditions such as psoriasis and eczema.

Morphoeic (sclerosing) BCC appears as a scar-like, waxy plaque or papule (Figure 34.4). The edges are not well defined, with tumour extension beyond the observed clinical margins. These usually occur on the face and can have ulceration, bleeding and crusting.

Histology

The histology shows neoplastic basaloid cells occurring in nests that are organised as islands of tumour cells more dense at the periphery (palisading) with a dermal inflammatory infiltrate (Figure 34.5).

Diagnosis

Clinical diagnosis is sufficient for most BCCs; however, if there is clinical doubt a biopsy is required. Superficial shave biopsy is the best diagnostic procedure for this epidermal lesion as punch biopsies risk introducing the tumour deeper into the dermis.

Treatment and management

• The age, symptoms, patient's general health and risk of the site (Table 34.1) of the tumour needs to be assessed before deciding type of treatment.

• Surgical excision is the most appropriate treatment for most BCCs. Larger lesions may require full thickness skin graft or flap repair depending on the site (e.g. face). Mohs' micrographic surgery is indicated in morphoeic BCCs for tumours with ill-defined margins especially if there are recurrent tumours at critical sites (e.g. eyelid or nose) (see Chapter 9). BCCs do not always require treatment. Curettage and cautery can be used for tumours located at low risk sites (e.g. trunk and limbs).

• Radiotherapy is useful for large tumours and elderly patients but the skin becomes atrophic and telangiectatic.

• Other treatments include cryotherapy for superficial BCCs (if multiple on the trunk), photodynamic therapy, topical 5-fluorouracil (Efudix®) and imiquimod 5% cream.

Prognosis

BCCs very rarely metastasise. Sun exposure is the major risk factor and sun protection is essential. There is a risk of recurrence if inadequately treated initially. A second BCC occurs in 20% of patients. Vigilance and early consultation regarding any new lesion is essential.

Squamous cell carcinoma

Squamous cell carcinoma (SCC) is the second commonest skin cancer arising from epidermal keratinocytes or appendages. SCCs can be locally invasive and can metastasise. Risk factors include long-term sun exposure, being elderly and having fair skin. SCCs occur on the ear, lip, hands and scalp, as indurated, crusted or nodular and ulcerated lesions (Figure 34.6). Tumours can arise *de novo* or within a previous solar keratosis or Bowen's disease.

Histology

Irregular nests of epidermal cells with normal and atypical dysplastic squamous cells are seen. SCCs can be classified as poorly, moderately or well differentiated tumours (Figure 34.7).

Treatment and management

- Management needs multi-disciplinary team input by dermatologists, plastic surgeons and radiotherapists. Full removal with histological confirmation of the primary tumour and any metastasis is needed. The type of SCC, location and risk of the site involved determine the overall treatment.
- Treatment of choice is surgical with either 3–5 mm margin excision (majority) or up to 1 cm excision margin (larger lesions) (Figure 34.8).
- Small, low risk lesions can be treated with curettage and cautery but radiotherapy and cryotherapy may also be used. Mohs' surgery may be required for ill defined and high risk lesions (Table 34.1), with radiotherapy after surgery for high risk SCC.
- Regular follow-up is necessary for 3–5 years after high risk SCC excisions to detect any recurrence at the original site or draining lymph nodes.

Prognosis

Primary cutaneous SCC has a good prognosis. Poorly differentiated tumours are more likely to metastasise. Large size and high risk site (e.g. lip and ear) worsens prognosis.

There is a 30% risk of having a second primary SCC within 5 years and immunosuppressed patients following organ transplants are more likely to develop multiple and more aggressive tumours. Patients with regional lymphadenopathy have <20% 10-year survival and those with distant metastases <10% 10-year survival.

Sun exposure needs to be prevented with sunscreens and protective clothing.

Keratoacanthoma

Keratoacanthoma (KA) is an epithelial tumour of hair follicle similar clinically to SCC. However, KAs grow rapidly over a few weeks and then spontaneously involute leaving an ugly 'moon crater' scar. A single nodule with central crater and keratin plug occurs on hair-bearing sun-exposed sites in the elderly (Figure 34.9). Full excision or incisional biopsy is required to exclude invasive SCC. Histology shows well-differentiated squamous epithelium with some cell irregularity with keratin formation centrally. Treatment usually surgical excision but also curettage and cautery, radiotherapy and cryotherapy are used.

Key points

- NMSC is increasing as a result of the increasing elderly population.
- BCC prognosis is excellent, with metastasis very rare.
- SCC prognosis is variable, depending on the histological differentiation and body site affected.

▶ Warnings

- High risk sites need to be treated urgently for both BCC and SCC.
- Mohs' surgery may be required to ensure complete removal.

Table 35.1

The American A, B, C, D system is:	The Glasgow seven point checklist consists of:

A = Asymmetry
 	
B = Border irregularity
 	
C = Colour variation
 	
D = Diameter >6 mm
	• **Major features:**
	  – change in size
	  – change in shape
	  – change in colour
	• **Minor features:**
	  – diameter 6 mm or more
	  – inflammation
	  – oozing or bleeding
	  – mild itch or altered sensation
	Note: lesions with any major feature or three minor features are suspicious of melanoma

Table 35.3 Main types of primary melanoma:

• Superficial spreading melanoma (80%) (see Fig. 35.6)
• Nodular melanoma (10%) (see Fig. 35.7)
• Lentigo maligna melanoma (5%)
• Acral lentiginous melanoma (5%) (see Fig. 35.8)

Table 35.2 Key features on dermatoscopy: (see Fig. 35.2)

• Asymmetry
• Number of colours
• Structure of the pigment
• Abruptness of the border

Fig. 35.1a/b Note mole larger and darker than others

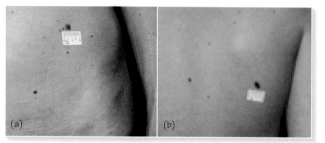

(a) (b)

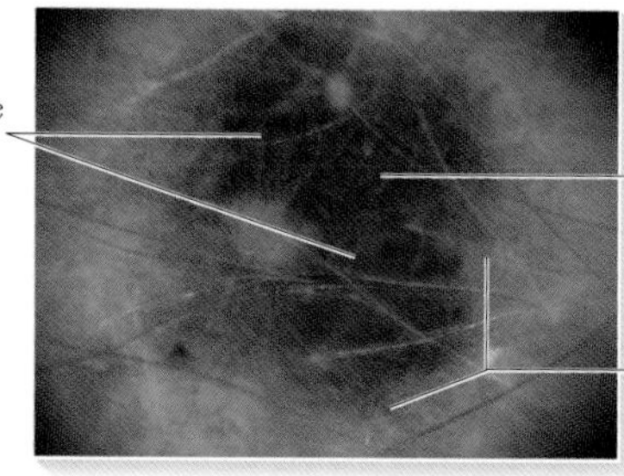

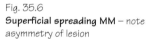

Variable colours

Fig. 35.2
Dermatoscope features
(see Table 35.2)

— Atypical pigment network

— Abruptness of border

Figure 35.3 Breslow thickness

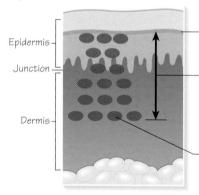

Epidermis —

Junction —

Dermis —

— Granular layer

— **Breslow thickness** determines prognosis by measuring depth of deepest melanoma cells

— Melanoma cells

Fig. 35.5
Note 1cm margin for excision

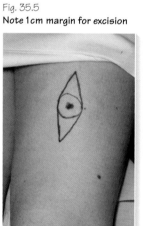

Fig. 35.6
Superficial spreading MM – note asymmetry of lesion

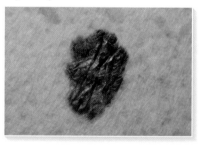

Fig. 35.8
Acral MM – note pigment in proximal nail fold

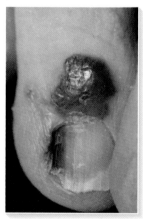

Fig. 35.4
Malignant melanoma pathology (H&E x40)

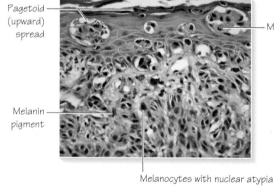

Pagetoid (upward) spread

— Mitosis

Melanin pigment

Melanocytes with nuclear atypia

Fig. 35.7
Nodular MM – note multiple colours and raised palpable areas

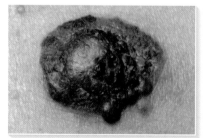

Dermatology at a Glance, First Edition. Mahbub M.U. Chowdhury, Ruwani P. Katugampola, and Andrew Y. Finlay.

Malignant melanoma (MM) arises from epidermal melanocytes. These tumours may arise within long-standing or new pigmented lesions. Melanoma occurs in any age in adults and can be unpredictable, with metastasis and death in a significant proportion of patients. Noticing an irregular pigmented lesion is key to early recognition and excision of a melanoma leading to the best opportunity for curative treatment.

Epidemiology

The incidence of melanoma has increased steadily. The incidence in the UK is around 10–15 cases per 100,000 population and has quadrupled in the last four decades. Thirty per cent of cases present at <50 years of age. Melanoma in childhood is extremely rare. Melanoma is the sixth most common cancer in women and the seventh in men. However, it is the second most common cancer presenting in the 20–40 year age group.

Malignant melanoma causes 80% of skin cancer deaths even though <10% of skin cancers are melanoma. More than 1800 deaths were reported in 2006 in the UK, with better survival rates in women because of thinner melanomas.

Risk factors

Risk factors for MM include exposure to sunlight (especially as a child and teenager) and UV exposure intermittently (holidays and regular sun bed use).
• Moderate risk factors: red hair, freckles and Celtic Caucasian skin type. Risk is 10–20 times lower in non-whites.
• High risk factors: increasing numbers of melanocytic naevi >6 mm in diameter, dysplastic naevus syndrome (atypical mole syndrome), family history of melanoma and large congenital naevi.

Melanoma risk has been linked with major genes including CDKN2A gene (chromosome 9), CDK4 gene (chromosome 12) and melanoma susceptibility gene (chromosome 1).

Diagnosis

Melanoma may arise in new moles, existing melanocytic naevi or congenital melanocytic naevi. There are a number of simple systems to aid clinical diagnosis of MM by naked eye inspection. The most common systems used are the American A, B, C, D rules and the Glasgow seven point checklist (Table 35.1).

The 'ugly duckling' sign is useful to remember. Any mole that stands out as being irregular compared with other moles present should always be treated with a high degree of suspicion (Figure 35.1).

Clinical examination is aided by a dermatoscope which allows closer examination of the surface of pigmented lesions with magnification and oil–glass interface or polarised light to reduce reflection on the surface. A score given can be correlated with the likelihood of malignancy depending on key features seen (Table 35.2; Figure 35.2).

Any suspected malignant melanoma lesion should be removed fully with primary excision with a 2-mm margin of skin followed by wide local excision, which reduces local recurrence. The local excision margins are determined by the Breslow thickness measuring the histological thickness of the tumour (Figure 35.3). For example, if the Breslow thickness is up to 1 mm then a 1-cm margin is taken. If it is more than 1 mm a 2-cm margin is taken.

An incisional biopsy may occasionally be warranted if a large lentigo maligna on the face or acral melanoma needs to be diagnosed. Other types of biopsies should not be used (e.g. shave and punch biopsies).

Pathology

The essential diagnostic pathological feature of melanoma is the presence of cytologically malignant melanocytes invading the dermis (Figure 35.4). The most common type is the superficial spreading malignant melanoma (SSMM) (Table 35.3).

Additional microscopic features include presence of ulceration, lack of maturation of dermal melanocytic cells, presence of lymphocytic infiltrate and atypical mitoses with angiogenesis at the base of the lesion.

The Breslow thickness measures the distance of the deepest invasive area of the primary tumour (in millimetres) from the epidermal granular layer. Lesions <1 mm thick are considered lower risk and >4 mm are higher risk. The Clark level can be measured on a scale of 1–5, with higher numbers indicating a deeper melanoma. Five-year survival falls with increased thickness of the tumour.

Management

Clinical diagnosis needs to be confirmed with histology and then definitive surgical excision with adequate clear margins (Figure 35.5). Dermatologists manage stage 1 and 2 MM as described in the 2001 American Joint Committee on Cancer (AJCC) staging system, where there is no lymph node or distant metastases involved.

Patients with intermediate, high risk or recurrent disease can have staging investigations including chest X-ray, liver ultrasound and CT scan of chest, abdomen and pelvis. Sentinel node biopsy or elective lymph node dissection is not currently a routine investigation and does not have proven benefit in improving clinical outcomes. Lymph node examination and appropriate treatment of draining lymph nodes are essential. Nodal disease and distant metastases may need palliative care.

Ipilimumab, a human anti-CTLA4 monoclonal antibody, has been shown to increase survival in patients with advanced melanoma.

Patients should be taught self-examination as early detection of recurrence is important.

Patients with invasive MM should be followed up 3 monthly for 3 years and discharged if <1 mm thickness. Thicker lesions >1 mm should be followed up for a further 2 years at 6-monthly intervals.

Prognosis

• For malignant melanomas of Breslow thickness <1 mm the 5-year survival is 95–100%.
• For 1–2 mm thick melanomas, 5-year survival is 80–96% and for lesions >4 mm thickness this drops to 50%.

Key points

• Malignant melanoma incidence is increasing.
• Malignant melanoma causes 80% of skin cancer deaths.
• Malignant melanoma with Breslow thickness <1 mm has a better prognosis.
• Always fully remove any suspected melanoma.

► Warning

Beware 'ugly duckling' sign to detect any irregular moles needing removal.

Fig. 36.1a/b Plaque and nodular stage CTCL on trunk

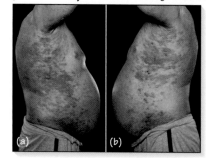

(a)   (b)

Fig. 36.1f Large ulcerating plaque

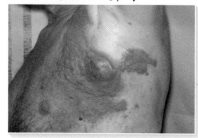

Fig. 36.1c Note atrophy and scaling

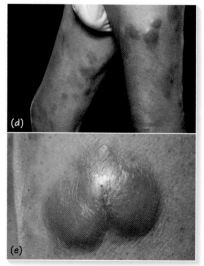

Fig. 36.1d/e Multiple nodules on legs and closeup

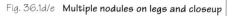

(d)

(e)

Fig. 36.2a Perianal Paget's disease

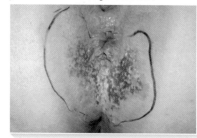

Fig. 36.3a/b/c
Kaposi's sarcoma on feet with closeup

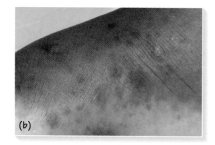

(a)

Fig. 36.4a/b
Metastases from
malignant melanoma

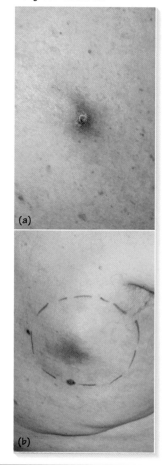

(a)

(b)

Fig. 36.2b Scrotal Paget's disease

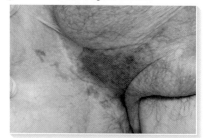

(b)

Fig. 36.2c Ulcerating Paget's disease

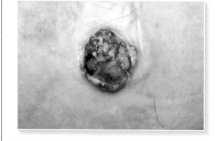

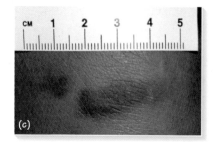

(c)

Dermatology at a Glance, First Edition. Mahbub M.U. Chowdhury, Ruwani P. Katugampola, and Andrew Y. Finlay.

Cutaneous T-cell lymphoma (mycosis fungoides)

Mycosis fungoides is the most common variant of primary cutaneous T-cell lymphoma (CTCL), a T-helper cell lymphoma of the skin. The cause is unknown. It has a male:female ratio of 2:1, with most patients diagnosed in their fifties and sixties.

CTCL can develop from patch stage to limited or extensive plaque stage and then tumour or nodular stage (Figure 36.1). The term parapsoriasis is used to describe a very early pre-diagnostic phase of CTCL. Multiple biopsies may be required over many years prior to definitive diagnosis.

Patients with CTCL present with ill-defined, red to pink scaly patches with atrophy and telangiectasia. The plaque stage consists of more red to brown elevated patches and plaques in the bathing trunk area affecting the buttocks, hip and upper thighs. Nodules that can ulcerate develop in the tumour stage. The majority have an indolent, slowly evolving disease but any form of CTCL may eventually invade the lymph nodes, peripheral blood and internal organs with a poor prognosis.

Sézary syndrome is a leukaemic form that can evolve from classic CTCL or develop with erythroderma (generalised scaling and exfoliative dermatitis). Pruritus and lymph node enlargement are common in Sézary syndrome.

Investigations include physical examination for lymph nodes and hepatosplenomegaly with a peripheral blood smear examination for Sézary cells.

T-cell receptor gene rearrangement (polymerase chain reaction and/or molecular studies) can be useful to identify monoclonal proliferation of T-cell clones in the skin. Renal and liver function, biopsy of enlarged lymph nodes, chest X-ray, CT scan and bone marrow biopsy may be required.

Histology typically shows superficial and deep band-like perivascular lymphocytic infiltrate with collections of lymphocytes (Pautrier's micro-abscesses) with thickened epidermis. The infiltrate is mixed with lymphocytes, eosinophils and plasma cells. Lymphocytes can be atypical with a hyper-convoluted or cerebriform nucleus (Sézary cells).

Differential diagnoses of CTCL include dermatitis, psoriasis and drug eruption especially in the erythrodermic form. The extent of the body surface area involved is important to document. In Sézary syndrome >5% of the total lymphocytes are CD4+ Sézary T cells.

Prognosis generally for the patch and plaque stage is good; however, more aggressive disease with spread to lymph nodes and organs, and also Sézary syndrome, have a poor prognosis.

Treatment options for early stages include emollients, potent topical corticosteroids and phototherapy (UVB, topical PUVA). Treatments for later stage disease include topical nitrogen mustard and oral bexarotene (a retinoid). Radiotherapy can be used for localised plaques or tumours. Sézary syndrome may warrant extracorporeal photophoresis. Treatments also include methotrexate, oral prednisolone and cyclophosphamide; however, chemotherapy is less effective.

Paget's disease

Paget's disease affecting the breast is a rare intraductal carcinoma presenting in the skin as a well-defined scaly patch or plaque which is eczematous around the nipple areola. This is often unilateral and can be confused with nipple eczema. Biopsy is essential. Extramammary Paget's disease is an intra-epidermal adenocarcinoma occurring more in women >40 years in the vulval area and perineum and in men in the scrotum, penis, anal and peri-anal skin (Figure 36.2). This usually develops as a grey, sharply demarcated plaque and may appear eczematous and thickened. Treatment includes local excision and radiotherapy may be needed for recurrences.

Kaposi's sarcoma

This is a malignancy of lymphatic and epithelial cells caused by human herpes virus 8 (HHV8). There are classic, endemic, transplant or HIV-associated types.
- Classic Kaposi's sarcoma (KS) is slowly progressive, occurring in 50- to 70-year-olds in the Mediterranean and Eastern Europe (Ashkenazi Jews).
- Endemic forms occur in Africa affecting children and young adults and can be more aggressive affecting the lower limbs.
- KS can occur in immunosuppressed patients, particularly in organ transplant recipients.
- AIDS-related KS affects the trunk, arms, head and neck and can be more aggressive involving mucosal surfaces. This has now reduced in incidence because of effective HIV treatment.

KS typically presents with small patches on the distal lower extremities which progress proximally (Figure 36.3). Lesions can become thickened and darker and the lower legs can become swollen and ulcerate. Fever, night sweats and weight loss can occur.

Skin biopsy shows neoplastic spindle cells with clefting and vascular channels. Differential diagnoses include malignant melanoma, pyogenic granuloma, CTCL or stasis eczema.

Treatment varies with the type of KS. Bigger lesions can be excised surgically. Multiple lesions require radiotherapy with chemotherapy. Immunosuppression-associated KS can improve with reduction in immunosuppression. HIV-associated KS can benefit from radiation, cryosurgery, intralesional vincristine and topical imiquimod.

Cutaneous metastases

These are uncommon and can be overlooked as a sign of underlying malignancy. Metastases present as firm painless subcutaneous nodules which can be indistinct. Skin biopsy confirms malignant cells of primary tumour origin and specific immunohistochemistry may be required for the final diagnosis. Prognosis is determined by the tumour type, extent of the disease and treatment options available. The most common causes are breast cancer, gastrointestinal cancer, melanoma (Figure 36.4) and tumours affecting the lung, kidney and ovary.

Key points

- CTCL is difficult to diagnosis and may require multiple biopsies over many years.
- KS may be an initial sign of HIV or AIDS related disease.
- Cutaneous metastases are rare but may indicate a poor prognosis. The three most common causes are breast cancer, gastrointestinal cancer and melanoma.

► Warnings

- New nodules arising in previous patch stage CTCL suggest transformation to a higher grade.
- Erythroderma with no previous skin disease should ring alarm bells. Perform a skin biopsy to exclude CTCL.

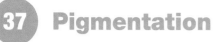

Table 37.1 Tanning

Protective mechanism against UV damage:

Three phases
1. **Immediate pigment darkening:** first few minutes after UV exposure, release of preformed melanin from melanocytes, rapidly fades. Induced by UVA
2. **Persistent pigment darkening:** lasts up to 24 hours. Induced by greater exposure to UVA
3. **Delayed tanning:** increased production of melanin first becomes visible after 2–3 days, lasts up to 2 weeks. Induced by UVB and UVA

Table 37.2 Tattoos (see Fig. 37.1)

Common phenomenon from early human history in all cultures, with strong cultural, social, religious and identity reasons for tattooing. May be accidental e.g. cycle accidents, grit from road

- **Risks of tattooing include:** infection (e.g. hepatitis from amateur tattooing), hypertrophic scarring or keloids, lichenoid reactions to red pigment, Koebner phenomenon at site e.g. in psoriasis
- **Treatment:** people change their minds about a tattoo, especially if a person is named or if a visible tattoo later reduces job opportunities. Localised excision is possible for small lesions. Laser therapy is most effective, though the skin does not become totally normal

Table 37.3 Drugs causing pigmentation

- Amiodarone: grey-blue changes in sun-exposed areas
- Minocycline: dark pigmentation of acne scars or diffuse pigmentation in sun-exposed sites (Fig. 37.9)
- Mepacrine: yellow
- Clofazamine: initially red, later blue-brown
- Localised hyperpigmentation in fixed drug eruptions e.g. co-trimoxazole, naproxen, tetracycline

Fig. 37.1
Tattoo with reaction to red pigment

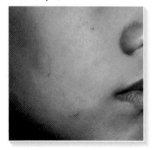

Fig. 37.2
Post-inflammatory hypo- and hyper-pigmentation from frequent rubbing

Fig. 37.3
Vitiligo of upper eyelid in child

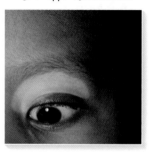

Fig. 37.4
Cheek with ill-defined pale areas of pityriasis alba

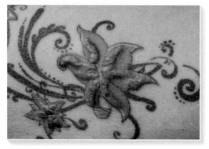

Fig. 37.5
Halo naevus – hypopigmentation around a mole

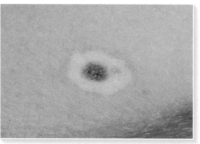

Fig. 37.6
Arms of child with oculo-cutaneous albinism between 'normal' arms

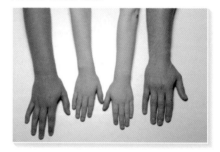

Fig. 37.7
Melasma affecting forehead of woman

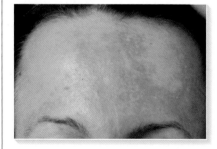

Fig. 37.8
Naevus of Ota – pigmentation involving sclera and around eye

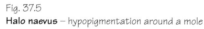
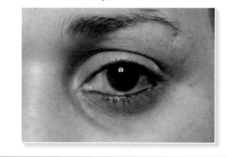

Fig. 37.9
Minocycline pigmentation of forehead

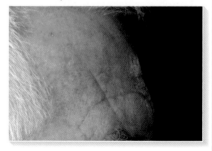

The visual impact of changes in pigmentation depends on the racial skin type. Vitiligo is more noticeable in people with dark skin and this is complicated by the cultural context: confusion with leprosy gives an extra stigma in some cultures, making it difficult for a woman with vitiligo to marry. Post-inflammatory hyperpigmentation is more obvious in darker skin, making it more important to treat inflammatory conditions such as acne effectively.

Effect of inflammation

Skin inflammation can cause increased (hyper) or decreased (hypo) pigmentation. Psoriasis plaques may leave pale areas after recovery that persist for years. Post-inflammatory hyperpigmentation can be severe if there is deep epidermal disruption (e.g. lichen planus). It follows the pattern of inflammation, which may be diagnostic (e.g. after herpes zoster). Pigmentation may follow trauma (Figure 37.2). Facial acne lesions can leave areas of increased pigmentation.

Skin lighteners
Lightening of skin colour

Reasons for desiring cosmetic skin lightening include cultural attitudes, a view that whiter skin is more attractive, and powerful influences from advertising by cosmetic companies. Medical indications for skin lightening include localised post-inflammatory pigmentation, treatment of solar lentigines and very widespread vitiligo if the normal darker skin appears abnormal. Reasons not to lighten skin colour include: natural skin colour is normal and attempts at lightening may not produce cosmetic benefit and may result in unnatural pigment variation.

How to lighten skin

Topical hydroquinone can be used alone, but it can be irritant and can cause irregular depigmentation. Hydroquinone is banned from cosmetics in Europe. Hydroquinone may be combined with topical tretinoin and/or topical steroids. Azaleic acid may be used. This chemical is produced by *Malassezia furfur* and causes the pigmentary changes in pityriasis versicolor.

Too little pigment
Vitiligo

Vitiligo affects 0.4% of the population (Figure 37.3). Flat symmetrical areas of depigmentation develop and enlarge. It is possibly caused by an autoimmune attack on melanocytes: they are absent from affected skin. It causes major psychological/social problems in some cultures or people with dark skin. Vitiligo is associated with pernicious anaemia, thyroid disease and diabetes.

Treatments include UVB or PUVA, potent topical steroids or melanocyte transplant from the same person. Melanocytes in hair follicles can multiply and repopulate surrounding skin. Patchy partial repigmentation may not be of perceived benefit to the patient.

Pityriasis alba

Areas of partial depigmentation and fine scaling develop (Figure 37.4) following mild inflammation, typically atopic eczema, on a child's face or limbs. Pityriasis means 'very small bran-like scales' and alba means 'white'. If any eczema persists, treat with topical steroids: normal pigmentation slowly returns.

Halo naevus

This is a white flat circular area around a benign mole, usually in children or teenagers (Figure 37.5). The mole may self-destruct in the autoimmune process that destroyed the surrounding melanocytes. Common and benign in children, so no treatment needed. It is rare in adults, suggesting malignancy: consider biopsy.

Oculocutaneous albinism

This is an autosomal recessive condition with absence or poor function of tyrosinase enzyme, essential for melanin production. Features include white skin (Figure 37.6), no retinal pigment, photophobia, nystagmus and squinting. In the most severe type (tyrosinase negative) there is white hair, pink skin and red eye reflex. If tyrosinase positive there is some pigment. Photoprotection is essential. Squamous cell carcinomas are frequent in tropical areas. In 'ocular albinism' the skin is normal.

Piebaldism

This is a rare autosomal dominant condition with white skin patches on the chest, abdomen and limbs and white hair at the front of the scalp (white forelock). Photoprotection is required.

Too much pigment
Melasma (also called chloasma)

Patchy increased pigmentation, often symmetrical, is seen on the face, especially the forehead (Figure 37.7), cheeks, above the lips and chin. It mostly occurs in women during pregnancy or on the oral contraceptive pill. Treatment includes sun protection and skin lighteners. Melasma gradually fades.

Incontinentia pigmenti

This is an X-linked dominant condition, fatal in males so only seen in females. In infancy recurrent small blisters and papules on trunk and limbs are seen. Blisters settle then hyperkeratotic lesions occur. Later whorled pigmentation persists with atrophic streaks. There may be defects of teeth, eyes and central nervous system.

Naevus of Ota and naevus of Ito

• **Ota:** brown–blue hyper-pigmentation one side of the face in trigeminal nerve distribution. There is hyper-pigmentation of the sclera of the eye (Figure 37.8).
• **Ito:** hyper-pigmentation over the shoulder, in posterior supraclavicular and lateral brachial cutaneous nerve distribution.

How not to mix up Ota and Ito: 'A in otA and in fAce, but I not in the eye.'

Argyria

Caused by chronic ingestion of silver, or absorption via lungs or mucosal surfaces, seen in silver mining, and manufacturing. Skin appears blue-grey, especially sun exposed areas. There is no treatment but the silver is non-toxic.

Key points

• Skin pigmentation is often altered by skin disease.
• Attempts to alter pigmentation may make matters worse, so first allow natural recovery.

► **Warning**

It is essential to ensure good photoprotection in vitiligo and albinism, to try to reduce the risk of skin cancer.

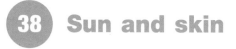

Table 38.1 **Clinical signs of photoageing**

- Coarse or fine wrinkling
- Coarsening of skin with yellow discolouration
- Skin fragility, scarring
- Deep wrinkles lateral to eye and mouth
- Erythema, pigment changes
- Telangiectasia, atrophy
- Comedones, milia

Table 38.2 **Sun protective measures**

- Physical and chemical sunscreens
- Clothing
- Hats and sunglasses
- Window protection e.g. car windows and home windows
- Stay indoors between 11 am–3 pm
- Umbrellas and parasols

Fig. 38.1a
Note irregular pigmentation, scaly solar keratoses

Fig. 38.1b
Marked wrinkling

Fig. 38.3a/b
Common sunscreens used with ingredients listed

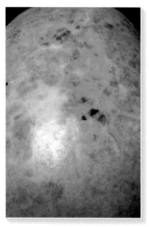

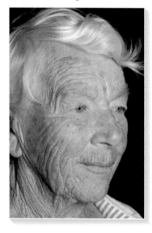

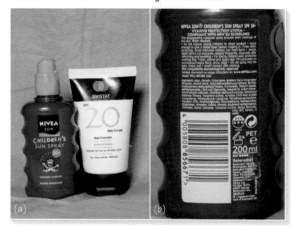

Fig. 38.1c **Photoageing comedones**

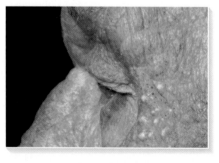

Fig. 38.4
Severe sun sensitivity requiring full body cover up with hat, scarf and gloves

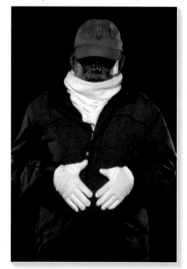

Fig. 38.2 **Note areas of normal skin tanning with vitiligo spared**

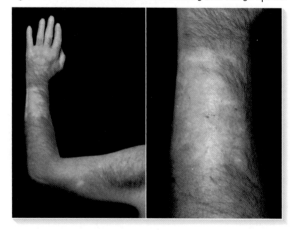

Dermatology at a Glance, First Edition. Mahbub M.U. Chowdhury, Ruwani P. Katugampola, and Andrew Y. Finlay.

The sun has many effects on the skin including sunburn, photoageing and tanning. The various responses to sun exposure depend on skin type and the ultraviolet light wavelength (see Chapters 39 and 40). The understanding of normal skin response to ultraviolet light is essential if abnormal responses are to be recognised. Fitzpatrick skin phototyping is most commonly used, from skin type 1 to skin type 6, based on assessing burning and tanning (see Chapter 39).

Sunburn reaction

The acute skin response to ultraviolet B (UVB) exposure is termed sunburn reaction and this is an acute inflammatory response.

Sunburn presents with painful erythema on the sites of skin exposure to excess UVB. Onset of sunburn can be delayed for 4–6 hours after sun exposure and can peak at 16–24 hours. It typically fades over 2–3 days and can be followed by severe peeling of the skin and tanning.

Sunburn is mediated by an acute inflammatory response that causes damage of the epidermal cells via cytokines and up-regulation of inflammatory adhesion molecule expression.

Photoageing

Photoageing or chronic sun damage is brought about by a gradual change in the skin structure and function following long-term recurrent exposure to sunlight or artificial ultraviolet radiation (UVR) sources. This is due to cumulative DNA damage from recurrent acute DNA injury and from the effects of chronic inflammation. Background intrinsic genetic ageing changes can also occur. The epidermis and dermis are affected mainly by UVB but the dermis is also affected significantly by UVA which can penetrate more deeply.

Clinical signs include cutaneous fine and coarse wrinkling, coarseness, dryness, telangiectasia with pigmentation, increased laxity with loss of skin elasticity and comedones (Table 38.1; Figure 38.1).

Skin types 1 and 2 are at greatest risk and photoageing signs may be apparent by the age of 40 years. The distribution is usually the face, neck and dorsum of the hands. Photodamage can progress even with attempted sun avoidance. It may also present with solar keratoses or skin cancer (see Chapters 34 and 35).

Treatment consists of topical retinoids such as tretinoin, alpha hydroxyacid or tazarotene. Skin peels (e.g. trichloroacetic acid) or phenol and laser resurfacing may be used. Surprisingly, the commercial product Boots No 7 Protect and Perfect reduces photoageing wrinkles in 20% of subjects after 6 months.

Tanning (Table 37.1)

Tanning ability varies with skin phototype: skin type 1 never tans and skin type 4 always tans (Figure 38.2). Tanning can be immediate or delayed and can occur within seconds of exposure to UVA. Immediate tanning results from photo-oxidative darkening and injury to epidermal melanocytic melanin. Delayed tanning of irradiated skin can persist for weeks to months and can appear over hours to days after exposure to all wavelengths of UVR. There is increase in melanocyte size mediated by tyrosinase activation and UVR induced melanocytic DNA damage. This leads to new melanin production. Tanning also varies with differences in UV exposure at different latitudes and heights.

Vitamin D synthesis

UVB radiation can convert epidermal 7-hydrocholesterol into pre-vitamin D3 which can then be isomerised to vitamin D3 and released into the circulation. Hence, sun exposure is an important step in the manufacture of vitamin D.

Limiting sun exposure has, in extreme cases, led to vitamin D deficiency in children. Sun exposure for 15 minutes 2–3 times per week should ensure adequate vitamin D levels in fair skinned individuals.

Sunscreens

It is essential to use sunscreens, particularly in photosensitive disorders, to protect the skin from further solar radiation causing damage (Figure 38.3). Sunscreens mainly block UVA, UVB or visible light or a combination. Sunscreens provide additional protection in combination with other measures such as hats, umbrellas, window protection and being indoors between 11 am and 3 pm (Table 38.2; Figure 38.4).

There are many sunscreens to choose from, which can be confusing. There are physical and chemical sunscreens.
- **Physical sunscreens** are usually opaque, containing titanium dioxide or zinc oxide and reflect UV radiation (UVA, UVB and visible light). These can look thick and messy on the skin but are more effective and so more protective against skin cancer.
- **Chemical sunscreens** absorb UV radiation, either UVA or UVB. UVB chemical sunscreens protect against UVB induced sunburn. The sun protection factor (SPF) indicates the UVB photoprotection in the sunscreen. SPF 10 means that after application, the person needs to stay out 10 times as long to reach the same level of tan or sunburn. Usual recommendations have been for 15–25 SPF for most patients but recent evidence suggests SPF 30 or higher is better. Cinnamates and oxybenzone in sunscreens can cause irritation or allergic contact dermatitis. The star rating (up to 5) indicates the UVA protection levels. Broad spectrum blocking sunscreens against UVA and UVB can be used.

Sunscreens need to be used liberally, thickly enough to cover the skin and evenly on all sun exposed skin areas including the lips, neck and ears. They need to be reapplied every 2–3 hours and after activities inducing sweating or swimming. Do not use sunscreens to prolong time spent in the sun.

To detect sunscreen allergy, the specialised test of photopatch testing is required (see Chapter 30).

Key points

- Both UVA and UVB exposure can cause long-term photoageing.
- Sunscreens need to be used regularly and in sufficient amount to have protective effects.
- Sun exposure leads to vitamin D production and avoidance of sun can lead to vitamin D deficiency.

▶ Warning

Sun exposure leads to photoageing which can be irreversible.

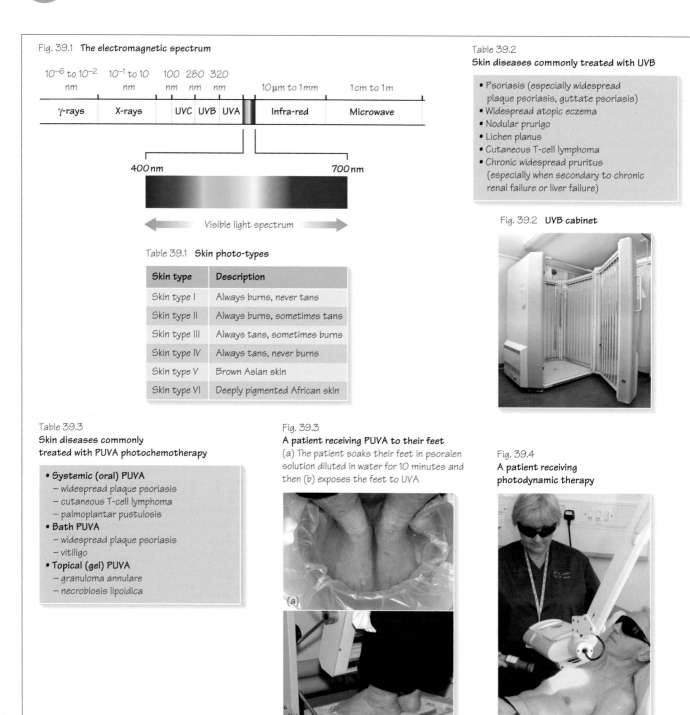

Fig. 39.1 **The electromagnetic spectrum**

10^{-6} to 10^{-2} nm | 10^{-1} to 10 nm | 100 nm | 280 nm | 320 nm | 10 µm to 1mm | 1cm to 1m

γ-rays | X-rays | UVC | UVB | UVA | Infra-red | Microwave

400 nm — 700 nm

Visible light spectrum

Table 39.1 **Skin photo-types**

Skin type	Description
Skin type I	Always burns, never tans
Skin type II	Always burns, sometimes tans
Skin type III	Always tans, sometimes burns
Skin type IV	Always tans, never burns
Skin type V	Brown Asian skin
Skin type VI	Deeply pigmented African skin

Table 39.2
Skin diseases commonly treated with UVB

- Psoriasis (especially widespread plaque psoriasis, guttate psoriasis)
- Widespread atopic eczema
- Nodular prurigo
- Lichen planus
- Cutaneous T-cell lymphoma
- Chronic widespread pruritus (especially when secondary to chronic renal failure or liver failure)

Fig. 39.2 **UVB cabinet**

Table 39.3
Skin diseases commonly treated with PUVA photochemotherapy

- Systemic (oral) PUVA
  - widespread plaque psoriasis
  - cutaneous T-cell lymphoma
  - palmoplantar pustulosis
- Bath PUVA
  - widespread plaque psoriasis
  - vitiligo
- Topical (gel) PUVA
  - granuloma annulare
  - necrobiosis lipoidica

Fig. 39.3
A patient receiving PUVA to their feet
(a) The patient soaks their feet in psoralen solution diluted in water for 10 minutes and then (b) exposes the feet to UVA

Fig. 39.4
A patient receiving photodynamic therapy

Dermatology at a Glance, First Edition. Mahbub M.U. Chowdhury, Ruwani P. Katugampola, and Andrew Y. Finlay.

Some skin diseases improve following sunlight exposure. Phototherapy is the use of ultraviolet radiation A or B (UVA 320–400 nm or UVB 280–320 nm) as a treatment (Figure 39.1).

Phototherapy: general principles

The skin response following exposure to UVA or UVB ranges from mild erythema or burning to blistering. 'Skin types' describe the tanning and burning response of individuals to natural sunlight as well as to phototherapy (Table 39.1). During life-long exposure to sunlight, UVA is responsible for skin ageing whereas UVB is responsible for sunburn. Prolonged exposure to natural or other UV radiation (sun beds, repeated phototherapy) can increase the risk of pre-malignant skin lesions and non-melanoma skin cancers. Patients who have received repeated courses of phototherapy should be educated and followed up to identify potential pre-malignant and malignant skin lesions.

Treatment is commenced with a dose of UVA or UVB that causes just visible erythema on that particular individual's skin (minimal erythema dose). The dose of UVA or UVB is then gradually increased depending on the clinical response. It is important to know what other treatment patients are taking during the course of phototherapy, as some drugs can make patients more photosensitive (e.g. tetracycline, amiodarone).

Phototherapy is considered as a second-line treatment option when topical treatments have failed, when a large body surface area is affected or where treating the individual lesions of the rash with active topical treatment is difficult as the lesions are small and widespread (e.g. guttate psoriasis).

UVB phototherapy

This is administered within a cabinet containing tubes emitting UVB at a pre-determined dose set by the operator (Figure 39.2). Narrowband UVB (311 nm) has replaced the previous use of broadband UVB phototherapy in many dermatology units.
- Skin diseases treated with UVB are listed in Table 39.2.
- Treatment is usually given three times a week up to a maximum of 20–24 treatments per course, depending on disease response. Some patients require repeated courses of UVB treatment during flare-ups of their disease (e.g. psoriasis); other conditions may require a longer treatment (e.g. cutaneous T-cell lymphoma).

UVA phototherapy

- UVA is given with psoralen, a photosensitising agent (PUVA). Skin diseases treated with PUVA are listed in Table 39.3.
- Psoralen can be given orally (in the form of 8-methoxypsoralen or 5-methoxypsoralen), or as 8-methoxypsoralen solution diluted in water for the patient to soak in for about 10 minutes (bath PUVA) or applied as a gel, prior to exposure to UVA.
- UVA is given in a phototherapy cabinet when a large body surface area is being treated, or in hand and foot PUVA units (e.g. for palmoplantar pustulosis) (Figure 39.3).
- PUVA can be administered with an oral retinoid (Re-PUVA) for the treatment of plaque psoriasis and palmoplantar pustulosis.

Important safely issues related to phototherapy

Prior to commencing phototherapy (UVA or UVB), patients are counselled regarding the treatment-related risks including skin malignancies and recommended the following safely precautions:

- Wear UV-protective goggles within the UV cabinet to minimise the risk of cataract. Patients having systemic psoralen should continue to wear UV-protective sunglasses for up to 24 hours post-treatment.
- Protection of genital area of men with appropriate clothing.
- Protection of non-treatment areas (e.g. use of visor for face).
- Photoprotection of skin on a long-term basis.
- Monitor for abnormal skin lesions by regular self-examination.

Phototherapy in special circumstances

- **Pregnancy and breast feeding**: UVB phototherapy is considered relatively safe in treating skin diseases during pregnancy and breast feeding (e.g. psoriasis, widespread atopic eczema). UVB phototherapy should be considered where topical treatments alone fail to improve the skin disease and systemic treatment is contra-indicated because of pregnancy or breast feeding.
- **Children:** the age at which a child is considered suitable for phototherapy depends on their ability to comply with the safety precautions within the phototherapy cabinet.

Photodynamic therapy

Photodynamic therapy (PDT) is a form of phototherapy that utilises high intensity visible light as opposed to ultraviolet light. PDT is used for the treatment of pre-malignant skin lesions (solar keratoses, Bowen's disease) and superficial basal cell carcinomas.

During PDT, methyl aminolevulinate cream, a photosensitiser, is applied to the lesion being treated and kept under occlusion for 3 hours. Selective uptake of the porphyrin precursor in this cream by the abnormal cells localises the treatment to the target area. After 3 hours, the cream is wiped away and the lesion(s) exposed to visible red light (570–670 nm) (Figure 39.4). This wavelength corresponds to the absorption peak of protoporphyrin IX, resulting in formation of highly reactive oxygen singlet species leading to localised destruction of the abnormal cells.

The common side-effects of PDT include pain during treatment and localised swelling, erythema, scabbing and, rarely, ulceration of the treatment area post-treatment.

> **Key point**
>
> - UVA or UVB phototherapy is a suitable second line treatment option for certain skin diseases where topical treatment has failed or when the disease affects a large body surface area.

> ▶ **Warning**
>
> Long-term risk of repeated phototherapy includes the risk of skin cancers. Patients receiving phototherapy should be counselled about this risk and educated to self-examine their skin to identify suspicious skin lesions.

Table 40.1 Classification of photodermatoses

	Immediate photosensitivity (trigger: visible light)	Delayed photosensitivity (trigger: visible and/or UV light)
Idiopathic photodermatoses	• Solar urticaria*	• Polymorphic light eruption (PLE) • Chronic actinic dermatitis • Actinic prurigo
Inherited	• Erythropoietic protoporphyria (EPP)*	• Congenital erythropoietic porphyria (CEP) • Xeroderma pigmentosa (XP) • Porphyria cutanea tarda (PCT)
Secondary causes		• Plants (phytophotodermatitis), e.g. contact with psoralen containing plants: rue, giant hogweed, celery • Drugs e.g. tetracyclines, amiodarone, thiazide diuretics • Metabolic e.g. PCT secondary to haemochromatosis or alcoholic liver disease

Table 40.2 Approach to a patient with a suspected photodermatosis

Clinical history
• Age of onset
• Seasonal variation in rash (worse in spring/ summer, improves in autumn/winter)
• Time interval between sunlight exposure and onset of symptoms and signs of skin disease
• Symptoms, e.g. skin burning/pain (EPP), itching (solar urticaria, PLE)
• Signs, e.g. no signs (EPP), urticaria (solar urticaria), papules and plaques (PLE), blisters (CEP, PCT)
• Family history e.g. XP, porphyrias
• Impact on daily activities and quality of life, e.g. restricted indoors, unable to do outdoor work and leisure activities
• Photo-protection measures
• Drug history, contact with plants, alcohol intake

Clinical examination
• Distribution of the rash: photodermatoses generally affect skin on exposed sites and spare covered sites
• Skin manifestations: e.g. scars and milia (EPP), blisters, photomutilation, hypertrichosis (PCT and CEP), marked freckling (XP)
• Morphology of lesions: e.g. phytophotodermatitis presents with linear erythema/blisters at the site of contact between the plant and skin (Fig. 40.1)
• Nails: photo-onycholysis (lifting of nail plate due to subungual blisters) noted mostly on finger nails
• Scalp: scarring alopecia due to recurrent blistering e.g. CEP

Investigations
• Serum auto-antibodies: antinuclear antibodies, extractable nuclear antigens, Ro and La antibodies, anti-double-stranded DNA antibodies
• Urine, blood and faecal samples for porphyria screen (samples need to be covered to protect from direct light)
• Monochromator light test
• Photopatch testing when a chemical or plant contact allergy exacerbated by sunlight exposure is suspected

Table 40.3 Classification of porphyrias

Main category of porphyria	Characteristic features	Examples

1. Cutaneous porphyrias:
  (a) Bullous
 	
  (b) Non-bullous
	Photosensitivity to visible light with:
	(a) Blisters hours to days after light exposure, milia, skin fragility, scarring, hypertrichosis
	(b) Skin oedema immediately following light exposure
		(a) Porphyria cutanea tarda (PCT)
		  Congenital erythropoietic porphyria (CEP, extremely rare)
		(b) Erythropoietic protoporphyria (EPP)

2. Acute porphyrias	Neurological and visceral features, e.g. peripheral neuropathy, abdominal pain, vomiting	Acute intermittent porphyria (AIP)
3. Cutaneous and acute porphyrias	Combination of the features of cutaneous bullous and acute porphyrias	Variegate porphyria (VP)

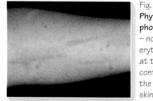

Fig. 40.1
Phyto-photodermatitis – note the linear erythema/blisters at the site of contact between the plant and the skin

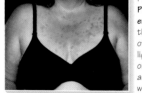

Fig. 40.2
Polymorphic light eruption – note the distribution of the rash to the light-exposed skin on the upper anterior chest wall

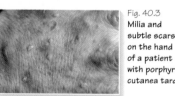

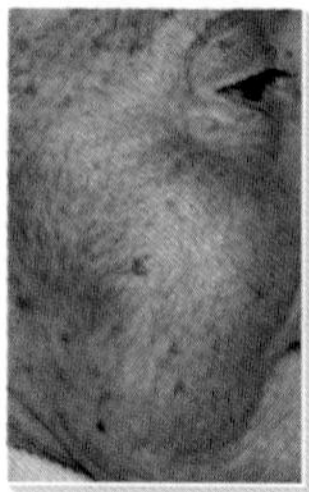

Fig. 40.3
Milia and subtle scars on the hand of a patient with porphyria cutanea tarda

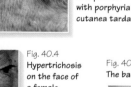

Fig. 40.4
Hypertrichosis on the face of a female patient with porphyria cutanea tarda

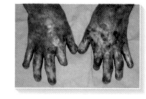

Fig. 40.5
Hands of a patient with congenital erythropoietic porphyria – note the blisters on the dorsum of the left hand, superficial ulcers due to burst blisters, severe scarring resulting in loss of finger nails, shortening of fingers and deformity of hands

Fig. 40.6
The back of a patient 24 hours following monochromator light testing

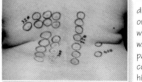

– the dark circles mark the sites of the different wavelengths that were shone on the patient's back. The erythema within some of the circles identifies the wavelength(s) that precipitated the patient's photodermatosis and helps confirm the diagnosis based on the history and clinical examination

Photodermatoses are skin diseases that are precipitated or aggravated by exposure to sunlight. They may be precipitated by one or a combination of different wavelengths of light: ultraviolet A (UVA 320–400 nm), UVB (290–320 nm) and visible light (400–750 nm). Photodermatoses can be idiopathic, inherited or secondary to other causes (Table 40.1). They affect exposed skin such as the face, anterior neck, upper chest wall, dorsum of the hands; photoprotected skin including behind the ears is usually spared (Table 40.2).

The onset of the rash following light exposure can be immediate or delayed. Patients with immediate photosensitivity usually present with an urticarial rash. Patients with delayed photosensitivity present with blistering, papules, increased freckling and/or eczematous rash.

Certain inflammatory skin diseases can be exacerbated by sunlight (e.g. rosacea, cutaneous discoid lupus erythematosus) or improved with sunlight (e.g. psoriasis).

Individuals with severe photodermatoses may develop vitamin D insufficiency or deficiency as a result of decreased sunlight exposure.

Polymorphic light eruption (Figure 40.2)

Polymorphic light eruption (PLE) is one of the most common photodermatoses, usually occurring at the beginning of spring and resolving by autumn. Itchy erythematous papules, plaques and vesicles on exposed skin appear about 1 day following exposure to bright sunlight.

Treatment includes sun protection (clothing, broad spectrum sunscreen) and moderately potent topical corticosteroids. Severe cases benefit from a 1-week course of oral prednisolone 20 mg/day at the onset of the rash. Narrowband UVB or psoralen plus UVA (PUVA) treatment at the beginning of spring can desensitise and 'harden' the skin to decrease the severity of PLE.

Solar urticaria

Itchy urticarial weals develop on sun exposed body sites within minutes of sunlight exposure. Lesions resolve within 24 hours. Solar urticaria is often precipitated by visible light, but UVA and/or UVB may also precipitate the rash. It may occur in association with PLE. Rarely, anaphylaxis may occur with bronchospasm.

Treatment includes sun protection (clothing, broad spectrum sunscreen) and anti-histamines. Gradual, cautious exposure to UVA phototherapy has been beneficial to 'harden' the skin.

Porphyrias (Figures 40.3–40.5)

Porphyrias are a group of inherited metabolic disorders. The individual porphyrias are caused by deficiency of the different enzymes involved in the haem biosynthetic pathway. The metabolites that accumulate upstream of the deficient enzyme lead to the manifestations of the individual porphyrias. The measurements of these metabolites in the patient's blood, urine and faeces aids in the diagnosis of the type of porphyria.

Based on the clinical manifestations, porphyrias are broadly divided into three categories (Table 40.3).

Treatment of all the cutaneous porphyrias is photoprotection from **visible light** with appropriate clothing and reflectant physical sunscreens that provide protection from both visible and ultraviolet light (as opposed to chemical sunscreens that only protect from ultraviolet light).

Porphyria cutanea tarda

Porphyria cutanea tarda is the most common cutaneous porphyria. It may develop from secondary causes such as alcoholic liver disease or haemochromatosis.

Treatment: regular venesection or oral hydroxychloroquine.

Erythropoietic protoporphyria

Patients require monitoring of liver function as they may develop liver failure necessitating a liver transplant. Patients with erythropoietic protoporphyria may benefit from oral beta-carotene to improve their tolerance to sunlight.

Xeroderma pigmentosa

This is a group of autosomal recessive diseases caused by defective DNA repair mechanisms.

XP is characterised by marked photosensitivity to sunlight, freckling and increased risk of multiple pre-malignant and malignant lesions of the skin (basal cell and squamous cell carcinomas, melanoma) and eyes from childhood.

Some 20–30% of cases may also develop neurological manifestations ranging from hyporeflexia to ataxia and quadriparesis.

XP is also associated with an increased risk of malignancies of the brain, lungs, kidneys, oral cavity and gastrointestinal tract.

Management includes diligent photoprotection, regular surveillance and treatment of pre-malignant and malignant lesions by a multi-disciplinary team. Oral retinoids have been used to decrease frequency of skin malignancies in XP.

Phototesting

Phototesting is used to detect the wavelength(s) of light that may provoke a particular photodermatosis. This is called monochromator light testing.

Light at different known wavelengths, which correspond to UVA, UVB and visible light, are shone on the patient's back. Evidence of localised visible erythema and/or skin oedema is checked immediately after and 24-hours post-irradiation (Figure 40.6).

Key points

- A rash in light exposed sites should raise the possibility of a photodermatosis.
- Photoprotection is essential in the management of all photodermatoses.

▶ Warning

- Phototherapy should be commenced cautiously in solar urticaria, as it may precipitate the rash and/or anaphylaxis.
- Patients with severe photodermatoses may require supplementation to avoid vitamin D deficiency resulting from decreased sunlight exposure.
- Numerous drugs can precipitate an acute attack of porphyria. The following website provides information on the safe use of drugs in acute forms of porphyria: www.wmic.wales.nhs.uk/porphyria_info.php

41 Skin signs of systemic disease

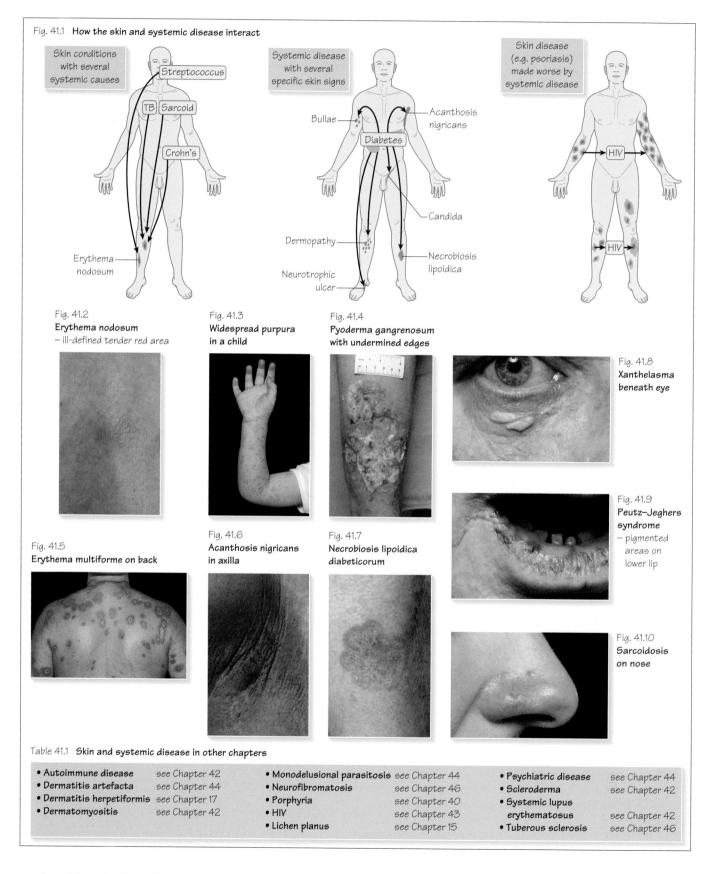

Fig. 41.1 How the skin and systemic disease interact

Skin conditions with several systemic causes
- Streptococcus
- TB
- Sarcoid
- Crohn's
- Erythema nodosum

Systemic disease with several specific skin signs
- Bullae
- Acanthosis nigricans
- Diabetes
- Candida
- Dermopathy
- Necrobiosis lipoidica
- Neurotrophic ulcer

Skin disease (e.g. psoriasis) made worse by systemic disease
- HIV
- HIV

Fig. 41.2
Erythema nodosum
– ill-defined tender red area

Fig. 41.3
Widespread purpura in a child

Fig. 41.4
Pyoderma gangrenosum with undermined edges

Fig. 41.8
Xanthelasma beneath eye

Fig. 41.9
Peutz–Jeghers syndrome
– pigmented areas on lower lip

Fig. 41.5
Erythema multiforme on back

Fig. 41.6
Acanthosis nigricans in axilla

Fig. 41.7
Necrobiosis lipoidica diabeticorum

Fig. 41.10
Sarcoidosis on nose

Table 41.1 Skin and systemic disease in other chapters

• Autoimmune disease — see Chapter 42	• Monodelusional parasitosis — see Chapter 44	• Psychiatric disease — see Chapter 44
• Dermatitis artefacta — see Chapter 44	• Neurofibromatosis — see Chapter 46	• Scleroderma — see Chapter 42
• Dermatitis herpetiformis — see Chapter 17	• Porphyria — see Chapter 40	• Systemic lupus erythematosus — see Chapter 42
• Dermatomyositis — see Chapter 42	• HIV — see Chapter 43	• Tuberous sclerosis — see Chapter 46
	• Lichen planus — see Chapter 15	

Dermatology at a Glance, First Edition. Mahbub M.U. Chowdhury, Ruwani P. Katugampola, and Andrew Y. Finlay.

It is not surprising that the skin is involved in many systemic diseases – it would be odd if it wasn't. Knowing about these clues to systemic disease is satisfying and gives you ('Sherlock Holmes') the chance of astonishing your colleagues with an accurate diagnosis on apparently little information.

Conditions with several causes

Erythema nodosum (Figure 41.2)
Ill-defined tender raised red lesions, several centimetres across, on the shins.
- Tuberculosis
- Sarcoidosis
- Beta-haemolytic *Streptococcus* – upper respiratory tract infection
- Drugs (e.g. oral contraceptive pill, sulphonamides)
- Autoimmune disease (e.g. systemic lupus erythematosus)
- Inflammatory bowel disease, especially Crohn's disease.

Pruritus (note correct spelling)
Generalised itchiness. First rule out skin causes of pruritus such as early pemphigoid, dermatitis herpetiformis or scabies.
- Hyperthyoidism
- Lymphoma (e.g. Hodgkin's disease)
- Renal failure
- Hepatobiliary disease, including cholestasis, primary biliary cirrhosis
- Iron deficiency
- Polycythemia rubra vera. Pruritus provoked by water contact (e.g. having a shower)
- HIV infection.

Purpura (Figure 41.3)
Red or dark blue areas, usually flat. Do not blanche on pressure because the red blood cells have come out of the blood vessels and are in the dermis.
- Low platelets (thrombocytopenia)
- Drugs (e.g. warfarin)
- Scurvy (vitamin C deficiency)
- Amyloidosis
- Henoch–Schönlein purpura
- Infections (e.g. meningococcal meningitis).

Pyoderma gangrenosum (Figure 41.4)
Persistent ulceration with purple undermined edge.
- Ulcerative colitis, Crohn's disease
- Rheumatoid arthritis
- Myeloproliferative disease (e.g. acute lymphoblastic leukaemia, chronic myeloid leukaemia, myelodysplasia, paraproteinaemia)
- Systemic malignancy.

Erythema multiforme (Figure 41.5)
Many red ('erythema') lesions over body and limbs. May be target-like but can be many shapes ('multiforme').
- Viral disease, especially herpes simplex
- Mycoplasma infection
- Drugs (e.g. sulphonamides), but many implicated.
Depending on the cause, withdraw drug or treat infection and provide urgent inpatient supportive therapy.

Acanthosis nigricans (Figure 41.6)
Dark velvety thickening in flexures, especially axillae, groin.
- Diabetes
- Insulin resistance and obesity
- Gastric adenocarcinoma.

Systemic diseases with specific signs

Endocrine disease
Diabetes
- Diabetic dermopathy. Atrophic brown scars on shins, thighs
- *Candida* infection
- Acanthosis nigricans (Figure 41.6)
- Diabetic bullae
- Neurotrophic ulceration
- Necrobiosis lipoidica diabeticorum (Figure 41.7).
This has a waxy yellow shiny appearance centrally and is typically on the shins. It indicates either the presence of diabetes or a strong risk of developing it. There is little evidence of effective therapy.

Addison's disease (adrenal insufficiency)
- Hyperpigmentation

Thyroid disease
Hyperthyroidism is associated with pruritus, pre-tibial myxo-edema and protruding eyes. In hypothyroidism there is dry skin with an ivory–yellow colour, coarse scanty scalp hair and enlarged tongue.

Metabolic disease
Hyperlipidaemia (Figure 41.8)
Xanthelasma (around the eyes) may occur with normal lipid levels but indicate increased risk of heart disease. Tendon xanthomas suggest familial hypercholesterolaemia and tuberous xanthomas (elbows and knees) suggest type III hyperlipoproteinaemia. Eruptive xanthomas (buttocks, back, limbs) indicate severe hypertriglyceridaemia.

Systemic cancer
Skin signs of systemic cancer are listed below:
- Cutaneous metastases (see Chapter 36)
- Tylosis (palmar keratoderma): oesophageal cancer
- Acanthosis nigricans (Figure 41.6): gastric adenocarcinoma
- Acquired ichthyosis (generalised stratum corneum thickening): Hodgkin's disease
- Dermatomyositis (proximal muscle weakness and mauve facial rash) (see Chapter 42): common systemic malignancies
- Erythema gyratum repens (waves of erythema reminiscent of the grain of cut wood): lung cancer
- Necrolytic migratory erythema (itchy red rash groin, lower abdomen, buttocks): glucagonoma (alpha cell tumour of pancreas)
- Migratory thrombophlebitis (Trousseau's sign): pancreatic carcinoma
- Acquired hypertrichosis lanuginosa (widespread excessive hair growth): lung, colorectal carcinoma.

Genetic diseases with skin signs and risk of systemic malignancy:
- Neurofibromatosis types 1 and 2 (see Chapter 46)
  - Malignant neurofibrosarcoma
  - Astrocytoma.

- Peutz–Jeghers syndrome (pigmented mucosal and skin macules and gastrointestinal polyps) (Figure 41.9)
  ○ Pancreas, breast cancer.
- Gardner's syndrome (subcutaneous fibromas, benign cysts, gastrointestinal polyposis)
  ○ Colonic cancer.
- Gorlin's syndrome (naevoid basal cell carcinoma syndrome)
  ○ Medulloblastoma.
- Tuberous sclerosis (epilepsy, mental retardation) (see Chapter 46)
  ○ Malignant sarcoma
  ○ Renal cell carcinoma
- Muir–Torre syndrome (sebaceous tumours)
  ○ Colonic adenocarcinoma (50%)
  ○ Urogenital malignancies (25%).

Systemic infection
Meningococcal meningitis: purpura.

Gastrointestinal disease
- Dermatitis herpetiformis (intensely itchy small blisters). There is gluten sensitive enteropathy associated with villous atrophy of small bowel and IgA anti-endomysial antibodies (see Chapter 17).
- Acrodermatitis enteropathica (blisters and scaling: perioral and acral [i.e. at end of limbs or fingers/toes]). Deficient zinc absorption leads to zinc deficiency.
- Liver cirrhosis. Signs include jaundice, pruritus, spider angiomas and body hair loss.
- Primary biliary cirrhosis. Associated with lichen planus (see Chapter 15) and hepatitis C infection.

Cardiology
LEOPARD syndrome
Lentigines widespread (brown flat areas), Electrocardiographic abnormalities, Ocular hypertelorism, Pulmonary stenosis, Abnormal genitalia, Retardation of growth, Deafness.

LAMB and NAME syndromes (Carney complex)
Lentigines, Atrial myxoma, Mucocutaneous myxomas, Blue Naevi, Atrial myxoma, Myxoid neurofibromas, Ephelides (freckles).

Important because identifies atrial myxoma which must be removed.

Sarcoidosis
Sarcoidosis (Figure 41.10) can be either primarily systemic or primarily cutaneous. Systemic sarcoidosis, typically with hilar lymphadenopathy, may present with erythema nodosum. Cutaneous sarcoidosis occurs as plaques, nodules or papules. Specific features include occurrence in scars (Koebner's phenomenon), red–blue swellings on ears or tip of nose (lupus pernio) and annular lesions especially on the face. There may be nail destruction with resorption of terminal phalanges. Diagnosis is based on skin biopsy, raised serum angiotensin-converting enzyme, chest X-ray and lung function tests. Therapy is with topical, intralesional or oral corticosteroids, or with chloroquine or hydroxychloroquine.

Key points

- Skin changes are often critical clues to systemic disease.
- The same pattern of disease can have several causes (e.g. erythema nodosum).

▶ **Warning**

Skin diseases may be altered by systemic disease. Pityriasis versicolor and psoriasis may become worse in HIV infection and viral warts may become worse on immunosuppressive drugs.

Table 42.1 **Classification of vasculitis**

- **Large vessel vasculitis:** giant cell temporal arteritis
- **Small/medium vessel vasculitis:** Wegener's granulomatosis, Churg–Strauss syndrome, polyarteritis nodosa, Kawasaki disease
- **Small vessel vasculitis:** Leukocytoclastic vasculitis, Henoch–Schönlein syndrome, cryoglobulinaemia and drug induced vasculitis, rheumatoid arthritis, systemic lupus erythematosus (SLE), Sjögren's syndrome

Table 42.2 **Causes of small vessel vasculitis**

- **Bacterial infections:** Streptococcus group A, Staphylococcus aureus
- **Viral infections:** Hepatitis, herpes simplex, fungal and parasitic infections
- **Drugs:** Penicillin, thiazides, quinine, oral contraceptives
- **Diseases:** SLE, rheumatoid arthritis, malignancies, capillary disorders, cutaneous T-cell lymphoma (mycosis fungoides), multiple myeloma, lung cancer, renal cancer, cryo-globulinaemia, ulcerative colitis, HIV infection

Table 42.3 **Tests to investigate vasculitis**

- Autoantibody screen (ANA, ANCA)
- Full blood count (normochromic anaemia, neutrophilia, eosinophilia)
- ESR, CRP
- Urea and electrolytes, liver function tests
- Chest X-ray
- Skin biopsy to show leukocytoclastic vasculitis
  e.g. Churg–Strauss syndrome is c-ANCA (cytoplasmic staining) positive and Wegener's granulomatosis is p-ANCA (perinuclear staining) positive

Fig. 42.1a/b **Discoid lupus erythematosus (DLE)** with scaly plaques and scarring alopecia on scalp

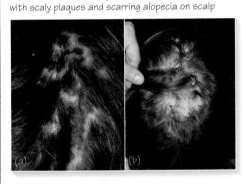

Fig. 42.1c **Note follicular plugging**

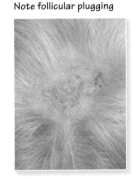

Fig. 42.1d **DLE on cheek with atrophy and scaling (closeup)**

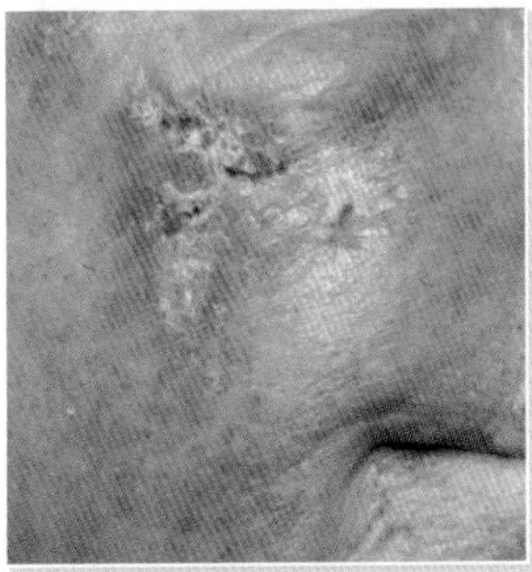

Fig. 42.2a/b **Subacute LE with annular patches on chest/arms**

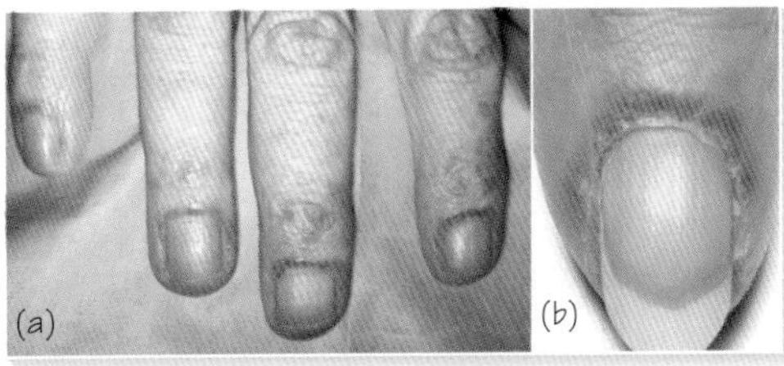

Fig. 42.3 **DLE**

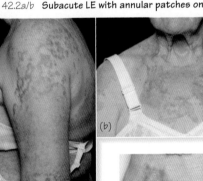

Fig. 42.2c **Subacute LE on dorsum hand**

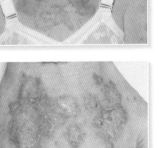

Fig. 42.4a/b **Nailfold capillary loops/ telangiectasia**

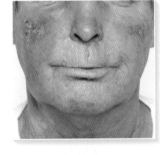

Fig. 42.5a/b **Sclerodactyly and calcinosis with closeup**

Fig. 42.6a/b **Heliotrope rash in dermatomyositis with closeup**

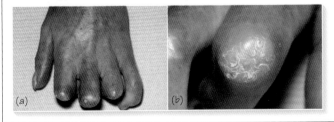

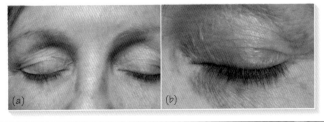

Dermatology at a Glance, First Edition. Mahbub M.U. Chowdhury, Ruwani P. Katugampola, and Andrew Y. Finlay.
© 2013 John Wiley & Sons, Ltd. Published 2013 by John Wiley & Sons, Ltd. **91**

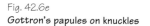
Fig. 42.6c/d
Rash in dermatomyositis on photoexposed areas *e.g. chest/arms*

Fig. 42.6e
Gottron's papules on knuckles

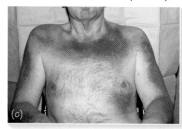
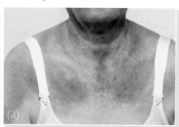
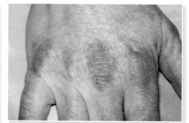

Fig. 42.6f
Gottron's sign on elbow

Fig. 42.6g
Gottron's sign on knees

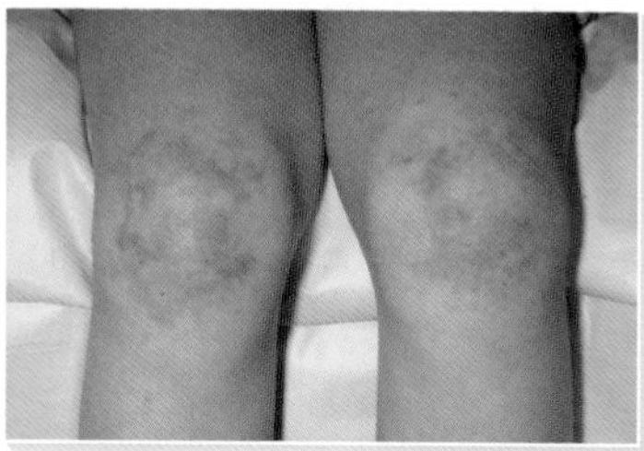

Fig. 42.6h
Nailfold changes and ragged cuticles with Gottron's papules

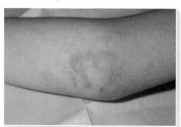
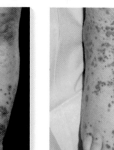
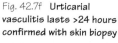
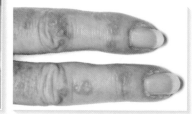

Fig. 42.7a Vasculitis with palpable purpura on legs

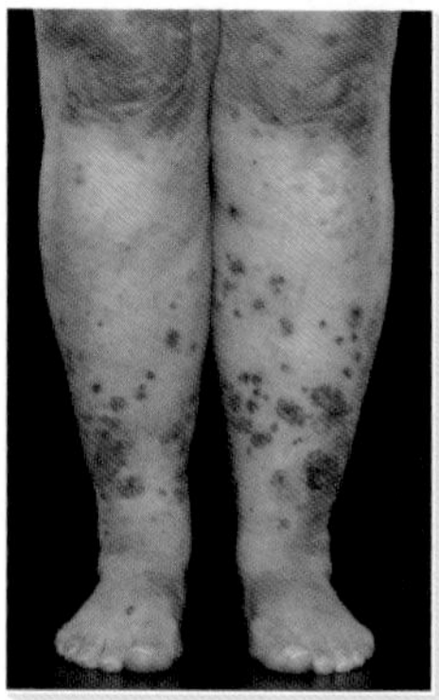

Fig. 42.7b/c Vasculitis on feet with closeup

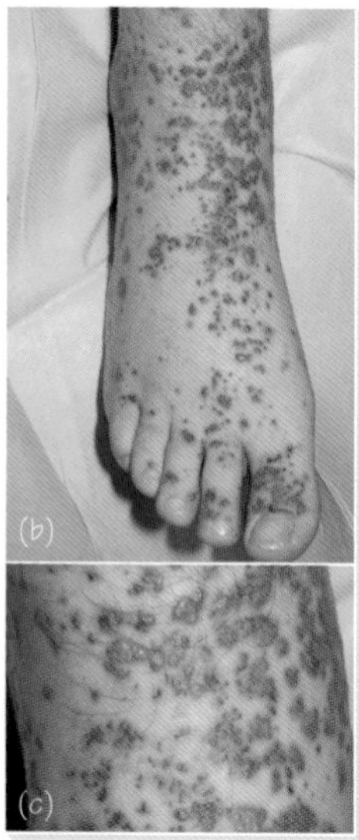

Fig. 42.7d Extensive vasculitis on buttocks

Fig. 42.7e Severe ulceration post-vasculitis

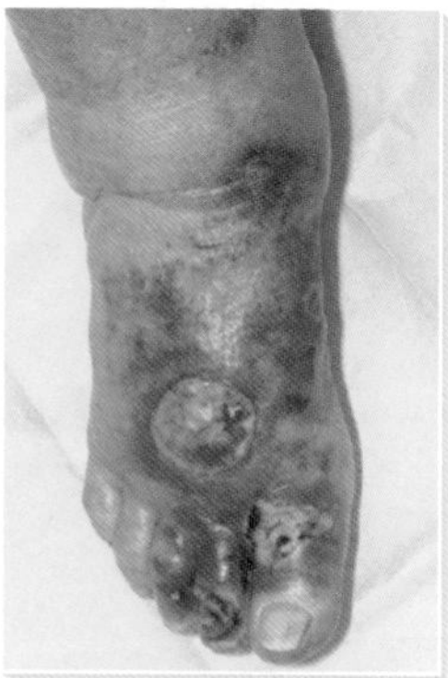

Fig. 42.7f Urticarial vasculitis lasts >24 hours confirmed with skin biopsy

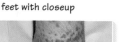
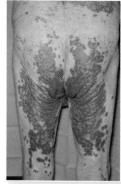
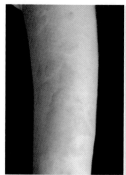

This chapter covers a broad range of diseases including lupus erythematosus, scleroderma, dermatomyositis and vasculitis.

Lupus erythematosus

There are many forms of lupus erythematosus with a wide range of manifestations ranging from localised chronic skin disease in discoid lupus erythematosus (DLE) to subacute cutaneous or systemic lupus erythematosus (SLE) with multiple organ disease. These diseases are thought to be caused by a variety of autoantibodies against cellular antigens including DNA, RNA and other proteins.

Treatment options include oral, intralesional and topical corticosteroids (potent to very potent), antimalarials (e.g. hydroxychloroquine) and dapsone.

Sunscreens are essential, with strict sun avoidance (see Chapter 38).

Discoid lupus erythematosus

This is the most common form with localised or widespread scaly red papules and plaques with central atrophy and scarring. DLE is more common in women with peak incidence in the forties.

Photosensitivity is present in 50% with 1–5% of cases progressing to SLE. The main sites affected are scalp, face and ears (Figures 42.1 and 42.3). Scarring alopecia can occur.

Clinical features include follicular plugging and adherent scaling with wrinkled epidermal atrophy. Lesions can be hypertrophic (thickened) leading to white or hyperpigmented depressed scars with telangiectasia.

Subacute cutaneous lupus erythematosus

This subtype has non-scarring red annular patches (Figure 42.2) or plaques in sun exposed areas on the upper trunk, neck, face and dorsum of hands. Photosensitivity is present in 70–90%.

Blood tests show positive ANA (anti-nuclear), anti-Ro (anti-SSA) and anti-La (anti-SSB) antibodies. Systemic involvement with kidney disease and leukopenia can occur.

Neonatal lupus erythematosus is a risk in affected women with transplacental transmission of antibodies (see Chapter 26).

Systemic lupus erythematosus

This is a multi-system disease affecting mainly women (8:1 ratio) aged 30–40 years.

Butterfly rash can occur (in 50% of patients) on malar areas of the cheeks and nose with red violaceous plaques or patches on the chest, shoulders and hands with scaling and follicular plugging. There is no atrophy and alopecia occurs in 20% of cases.

Skin biopsy is needed for histology and immunofluorescence with autoantibody screen of blood to confirm positive ANA and anti-double-stranded DNA.

Other manifestations include fever, arthritis, vasculitis, Raynaud's phenomenon, oral mucosal ulceration and nail fold capillary changes with prominent capillary loops (Figure 42.4), and renal, cardiac, lung and nervous system abnormalities.

Scleroderma (systemic sclerosus)

This is an idiopathic condition causing diffuse or localised fibrosis. The diffuse form can have internal organ fibrosis and vascular abnormalities.

CREST syndrome is a localised form with **C**alcinosis, **R**aynaud's disease, o**E**sophageal dysmotility, **S**clerodactyly and **T**elangiectasia. This most commonly involves the hands (Figure 42.5) and face. This occurs mainly in women (3:1 ratio) with peak onset at 30–50 years.

Skin changes include smooth shiny pigmented indurated skin with restricted mouth opening, perioral puckering, Raynaud's phenomenon, facial telangiectasia, sclerodactyly, dilated nail fold capillaries with ragged cuticles, calcinosis cutis (Figure 42.5b) and livedo reticularis. Fingertip ulceration and gangrene is common and diffuse calcification of the skin may occur.

Tests to confirm diagnosis include positive ANA (90%) with nucleolar pattern staining, antibodies to Scl70 and anti-centromere antibodies (highly specific for CREST syndrome).

No treatment reverses fibrosis of the skin. Raynaud's phenomenon is treated with calcium channel blockers. Cessation of smoking can improve digital ulceration and resistance to trauma.

Dermatomyositis

This is an idiopathic connective tissue disease which may be linked with underlying malignancy (paraneoplastic) especially in the elderly. Fatigue, proximal symmetrical muscle weakness and dysphagia can occur.

Skin features (Figure 42.6) include a peri-orbital heliotrope (blue–purple colour) rash (Figure 42.6a,b), Gottron's papules (red plaques on extensor finger joints) (Figure 42.6e), erythema over knees and elbows (Gottron's sign) (Figure 42.6f,g), dilated nail fold capillaries and ragged cuticles (Figure 42.6h). Ten per cent of patients have skin findings without muscle disease (amyopathic dermatomyositis).

Serum creatinine kinase is usually raised and a muscle biopsy may be required. Anti-Jo-1 antibody positive (20%) is associated with interstitial lung disease and arthritis.

The disease course may progress or remit spontaneously.

Treatments include sun protection, systemic corticosteroids, hydroxychloroquine and steroid-sparing agents (e.g. methotrexate, azathioprine).

Screening tests for underlying malignancy should be carried out.

Small vessel vasculitis

Vasculitis can be classified as caused by inflammation in specific blood vessel walls (Table 42.1). In 60% of patients no cause is found, in others there is deposition of IgG or IgM immune complexes in post-capillary venules.

The principal skin sign is palpable purpura which can be painful. Skin signs include livedo reticularis (a blotchy net-like pattern), purpura, erythema multiforme and urticaria. These signs occur on dependent areas on the back, buttocks and lower legs (Figure 42.7).

Vasculitis can be caused by infection, drugs, food allergy, connective tissue diseases and malignancy (Table 42.2). A full vasculitis screen (Table 42.3) includes full blood count, renal and liver function, autoantibody screen (ANA, anti-neutrophil cytoplasmic antibody [ANCA]), ESR, chest X-ray and skin biopsy to show leukocytoclastic vasculitis.

Patients with systemic vasculitis can present with malaise, fever, weight loss and glomerulonephritis, sensory neuropathy, abdominal pain and haemorrhage, angina and stroke.

Prognosis is dependent on factors such as renal involvement. The condition resolves within a few weeks if precipitating factors can be removed. NSAIDs can be used for general symptoms and systemic steroids (60–80 mg/day) with other immunosuppressive agents can help (e.g. cyclophosphamide, methotrexate, azathioprine or ciclosporin).

Key points

- All forms of lupus erythematosus need strict sun avoidance.
- Think widely for causes of vasculitis including drugs, infections and systemic diseases.

► Warning

Suspected vasculitis should be urgently investigated and treated.

Figure 43.1 **Manifestations of HIV**

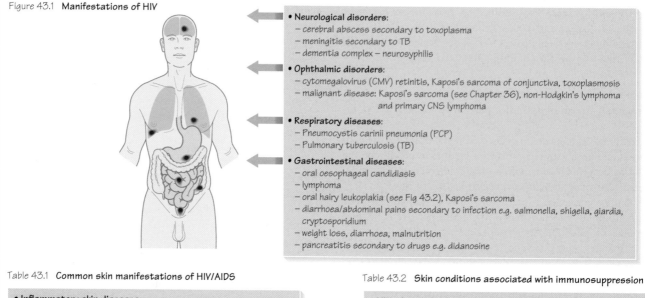

- **Neurological disorders:**
  - cerebral abscess secondary to toxoplasma
  - meningitis secondary to TB
  - dementia complex – neurosyphilis
- **Ophthalmic disorders:**
  - cytomegalovirus (CMV) retinitis, Kaposi's sarcoma of conjunctiva, toxoplasmosis
  - malignant disease: Kaposi's sarcoma (see Chapter 36), non-Hodgkin's lymphoma and primary CNS lymphoma
- **Respiratory diseases:**
  - Pneumocystis carinii pneumonia (PCP)
  - Pulmonary tuberculosis (TB)
- **Gastrointestinal diseases:**
  - oral oesophageal candidiasis
  - lymphoma
  - oral hairy leukoplakia (see Fig 43.2), Kaposi's sarcoma
  - diarrhoea/abdominal pains secondary to infection e.g. salmonella, shigella, giardia, cryptosporidium
  - weight loss, diarrhoea, malnutrition
  - pancreatitis secondary to drugs e.g. didanosine

Table 43.1 **Common skin manifestations of HIV/AIDS**

- **Inflammatory skin diseases:**
  Psoriasis, eczema, seborrhoeic dermatitis (Fig. 43.3), folliculitis
- **Infections:**
  - viral: herpes zoster/herpes simplex, CMV, molluscum contagiosum (Fig. 43.5), human papilloma virus (HPV)
  - fungal: Malassezia, Cryptococcus, Histoplasma, Candida
  - bacterial: TB, syphilis, bacillary angiomatosis
- **Problems due to drugs:**
  - Stevens-Johnson syndrome: cotrimoxazole, nevirapine, efavirenz
  - nail pigmentation: indinavir, zidovudine, ritonavir
  - lipodystrophy: indinavir, ritonavir
- **Malignancy:**
  - Kaposi's sarcoma (Fig. 43.4), lymphoma

Table 43.2 **Skin conditions associated with immunosuppression**

- HIV related skin conditions (see Table 43.1)
- Skin cancer in transplant recipients (see Chapter 34)
- Molluscum contagiosum
- Melanoma/SCC/BCC (see Chapters 35 and 34)
- Skin lymphoma (see Chapter 36)
- Varicella zoster, herpes simplex infections (see Chapter 19)
- Warts e.g. common viral wart, HPV (see Chapter 19)

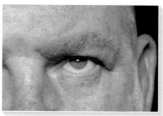

Fig. 43.3
Seborrhoeic dermatitis affecting eyebrows

Fig. 43.2a/b Oral hairy leukoplakia on lateral tongue border

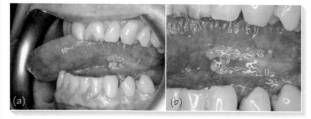

Fig. 43.4a/b
Kaposi's sarcoma on sole showing patch and nodule, with closeup

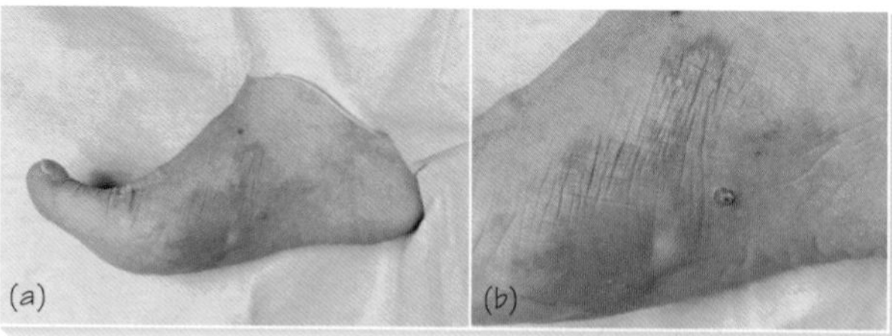

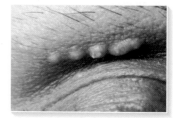

Fig. 43.5a
Typical molluscum

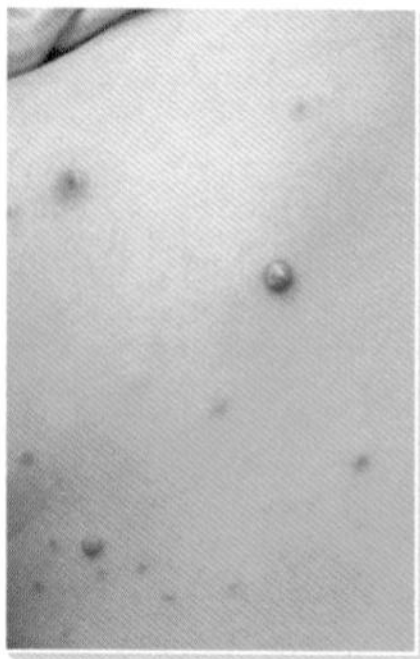

Fig. 43.5b
Widespread molluscum in HIV

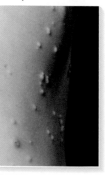

Fig. 43.5c
Note central dimples in papules

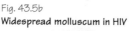

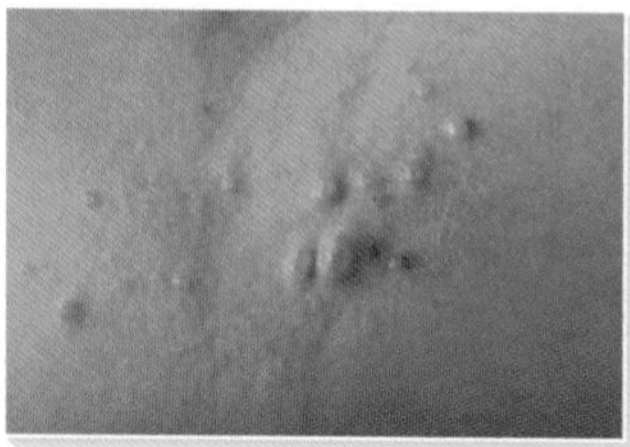

Fig. 43.5d
Molluscum on upper eyelid after topical steroid use

Dermatology at a Glance, First Edition. Mahbub M.U. Chowdhury, Ruwani P. Katugampola, and Andrew Y. Finlay.

Immunosuppressed patients are prone to infections and skin cancers. This chapter covers HIV infection and skin conditions seen in immunocompromised patients.

Human immunodeficiency virus infection

Over 30 million people are infected with HIV and 65% of these are in sub-Saharan Africa. In the UK around 60,000 individuals are affected. There are around 6000 new cases per year with 10% presenting with advanced HIV disease or AIDS (acquired immunodeficiency syndrome).

The HIV virus is transmitted by sexual intercourse, contaminated injections used by drug abusers, blood products, breast milk and by perinatal transmission. This can co-exist with other sexually transmitted infections such as hepatitis C.

HIV is a human retrovirus containing RNA which transcribes DNA via a reverse transcriptase enzyme. HIV infection leads to CD4 cell depletion starting as a primary cell immunity defect progressing to general immune dysfunction. A CD4 count of $<200 \, mm^2$ (normal $>500 \, mm^2$) is regarded as diagnostic of AIDS. Markers of disease progression include high HIV viral load measured by polymerase chain reaction (PCR) assay. These markers can also be used to monitor response to treatment.

HIV seroconversion (HIV p24 antigen detectable) can occur up to 3 months after infection. Twenty-five per cent develop clinical seroconversion illness consisting of fever, malaise, rash, sore throat, lymphadenopathy and arthralgia. HIV PCR and p24 antigen confirm the diagnosis of HIV and an antibody test (Western blot or immunofluorescence assay) can also be carried out.

The Centers for Disease Control and Prevention (CDC) classification stages the disease from primary seroconversion illness through to AIDS related complex (advanced HIV disease with opportunistic infection or tumours) (Figure 43.1).

Skin manifestations of HIV/AIDS can affect up to 75% of HIV patients (Table 43.1). The acute HIV illness can present with an asymptomatic macular or papular rash affecting the face and trunk and also seborrhoeic dermatitis (Figure 43.3).

All skin diseases and other infections can be atypical and more persistent and severe than usual, often responding poorly to standard treatment. If this occurs with any common conditions such as psoriasis and seborrhoeic dermatitis, HIV screening should be considered at an early stage.

Highly active anti-retroviral treatment regimen (HAART) involves three drug combinations to suppress viral replication and to reduce the risk of viral resistance. Prognosis is predicted by viral resistance as well as factors such as drug tolerance, side effects and adherence (i.e. compliance). Drugs used include nucleoside reverse transcriptase inhibitors (zidovudine, didanosine), protease inhibitors (ritonavir, indinavir, saquinavir) or non-nucleoside reverse transcriptase inhibitors (efavirenz, nevirapine). Twenty-five per cent of hospital admissions with HIV are a result of drug side effects (Table 43.1).

Generalised macular and papular rashes are common with co-trimoxazole and nevirapine. Nevirapine and efavirenz can cause Stevens–Johnson syndrome or toxic epidermal necrolysis.

Prognosis was markedly improved with the introduction of HAART therapy in 1997 and death rates have reduced for those aged 25–40 years. Opportunistic illnesses have reduced except lymphoma which is increasing in incidence.

Immune reconstitution inflammatory syndrome (IRIS) may be triggered by HAART therapy and skin conditions can develop when CD4 and CD8 counts increase (e.g. herpes and viral wart infections, Kaposi's sarcoma (Figure 43.4) and eosinophilic folliculitis).

Immunocompromised patients and skin conditions

Any immunocompromised patient can be more prone to skin problems. Therapies such as oral tacrolimus, azathioprine, ciclosporin and mycophenolate mofetil may predispose to skin tumours and skin infections. The commonly associated conditions are listed in Table 43.2.

Skin cancer in immunosuppressed transplant recipients can be more aggressive with early recurrences and metastases. Therapy to ensure full surgical removal is needed.

In some centres regular monitoring of transplant patients for skin cancers may be undertaken ensuring increased vigilance at follow-up.

Types of skin cancers that may be more common include squamous cell carcinoma, melanoma and basal cell carcinoma (see Chapters 34 and 35).

Key points

- Always consider HIV infection if skin conditions are severe, atypical and less responsive to standard treatments.
- Drug therapy for HIV infection may cause skin problems including dermatological emergencies such as Stevens–Johnson syndrome or toxic epidermal necrolysis.
- Immunosuppressed patients present with a wide range of common skin conditions which may be more severe and persistent (e.g. viral warts).

► Warning

Skin cancers in immunosuppressed transplant patients may be more aggressive and metastasise early. Full surgical clearance of the tumour and close monitoring is required.

Table 44.1 Skin disease aggravated/provoked by psychological problems

- **Alopecia areata**
  Severe stress can result in hair loss (alopecia areata). Before the Battle of Corruna (1809) General Sir John Moore's hair turned white: typically in alopecia areata the dark hairs are shed more easily
- **Psoriasis**
  Many patients feel that their psoriasis started or became worse after stressful events such as a family death or financial problems. Stress may affect cortisol levels and provoke increased psoriasis severity
- **Atopic eczema**
  Adult atopic eczema is associated with depression, stress-related and behavioural disorders. It is difficult to separate out which aspects of behaviour are caused by the disease, and which by personality

Fig. 44.1 Mind–skin–interpersonal interaction

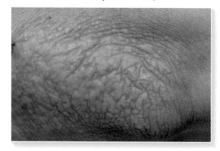

I'm worried about how she'll react to my skin

Is it catching? It looks horrible

Skin disease impact on mind

Psychological outlook impact on skin disease

Fig. 44.2 Dermatitis artefacta – ulcers

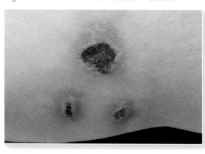

Fig. 44.4 How itch leads to nodular prurigo

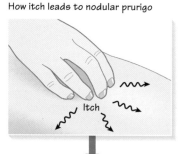

Itch

Scratch

Calendar
1 2 3 4 5 6 7
8 9 10 11 12 13 14

Lichen simplex

Calendar
Mar Apr May

Nodular prurigo

Fig. 44.3 Factitial purpura, caused by sucking on a glass

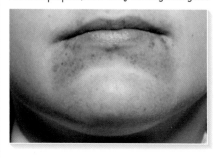

Fig. 44.5 Lichen simplex on elbow
– thickening after frequent rubbing

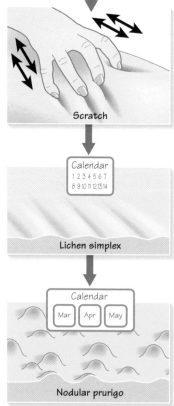

Fig. 44.6 Nodular prurigo with excoriations

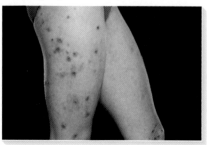

Dermatology at a Glance, First Edition. Mahbub M.U. Chowdhury, Ruwani P. Katugampola, and Andrew Y. Finlay.

Skin disease often results in psychological problems. As the skin is so visible and because it has such a major role in formal and intimate communication, relationships may be impaired and self-esteem lowered, resulting in distress that may be hard to resolve (Figure 44.1). The prevalence of depression is high in people with widespread skin disease; this is often unrecognised by their carers. Therefore, it is important in all patients to consider their psychological state, especially in chronic widespread inflammatory skin disease (Table 44.1). There are a few skin diseases in which psychological influences or mental illness have a major causative role.

Psychiatric and skin co-morbidity

• Depression: high prevalence in severe psoriasis.
• Obsessive–compulsive disorder (OCD): may cause excessive scratching in atopic dermatitis. Hand dermatitis occurs with frequent hand washing.
• Social phobia: anxious avoidance of social situations where previously their skin condition resulted in problems.
• Body dysmorphic disorder: distorted self-image.

Skin diseases primarily caused by psychological and psychiatric problems

Factitious dermatitis

Rarely, people deliberately damage their skin, sometimes repeatedly over many months or years. They draw attention to the damaged skin and seek treatment, but deny any knowledge of how it was caused: both lesions and history are false. They may cause non-healing ulcers by constantly picking at the skin (Figure 44.2), by injecting toxic matter or by cigarette burns. Lesions may be odd shapes (Figure 44.3). Patients may gain by taking on a sickness role.

Management is very difficult. Clearly, the patient needs psychological help. It is debatable whether it is helpful to confront a patient with the diagnosis. A face-saving strategy is to allow the patient to retreat from the self-harming procedure without having to admit their responsibility for it.

Delusional infestation (parasitosis)

This is a monodelusion, a psychiatric disorder with a single focus in a person who otherwise functions normally. Patients become unshakeably convinced that they are infested, usually by an insect or parasite. They convince friends and family of this and their partners may become convinced that they are also infested (folie à deux). Typically, they will bring in a small piece of matter that they claim is a parasite that they have squeezed out of their skin: invariably under the microscope there is no evidence of any parasite. Patients 'doctor shop', and often complain about their care, as they are convinced that they are 'infected' and do not accept that they have a psychiatric problem. Often homes have been fumigated after others have taken the patient's complaint at face value.

Management involves reaching an agreement with the patient that they have a problem (unspecified) that needs solving and prescribing second generation anti-psychotics, e.g. olanzapine.

'Morgellons' syndrome' is a descriptor now self-adopted by many patients whom most dermatologists and psychiatrists believe have monodelusional infestation. The popularity of this new descriptor is an interesting phenomenon in itself. The internet now allows people with psychological problems to communicate in a way previously impossible. This may have many benefits, especially for mutual support, but here seems to have resulted in an ongoing 'folie à mille'.

Dysmorphic disorder

Most people have an inaccurate self-perception of how they look to others: for example, medical students when watching a video recording of themselves in a clinic may be surprised at how they appear. However, some people's self-perception is so widely distorted that their behaviour is inappropriately affected. Body dysmorphic disorder may focus on different body aspects, such as weight or skin. A very small amount of physiological acne, barely visible to even a close observer, may be perceived as of huge significance and be blamed by the patient for problems in their life. The doctor's difficulty in not being able to see what the patient is concerned about resulted in the term 'dermatological non-disease'.

Patients may insist on powerful systemic therapy or on cosmetic procedures that do not appear to be indicated. Often, any procedure carried out does not satisfy the patient, with risks of complaints and litigation. There may be an association with OCD and there is a risk of suicide.

Management requires reaching agreement with the patient that there is distress and disability, and considering cognitive behaviour therapy or use of specific serotonin reuptake inhibitors.

Damaging habits
Trichotillomania

There is shortening or baldness of scalp hair caused by the patient deliberately pulling individual hairs out. Children often deny doing this. A major clue is that the hairs in the affected area are usually of different lengths. In a child this is a sign of psychological distress but in an adult it may be a more serious sign of psychiatric disease.

Neurodermatitis

If you have itchy skin it is very difficult not to scratch (Figure 44.4) and current therapies for itch are not very effective. Repeated scratching results in damage to the skin, 'neurodermatitis'. To begin with there is superficial damage to the skin, 'excoriations' (scratches). Repeated trauma induces the skin protective mechanism of thickening, resulting in 'lichen simplex' (Figure 44.5). This is itchy itself, so the scratching and rubbing continue, eventually resulting in a lumpy or cobblestone appearance, 'nodular prurigo' (Figure 44.6). The underlying skin disease is treated and topical steroids applied to the inflammatory changes, along with antibiotics if there are signs of secondary bacterial infection. Protection of the skin with occlusive bandages (where possible) is the single most useful technique, in order to break the vicious itch–scratch cycle.

> ### Key point
> • Educational and psychological training programmes can improve the quality of life of patients with chronic skin disease.

> ### ► Warning
> There is a suicide risk in body dysmorphic disorder: don't dismiss it.

Table 45.1 **Causes of leg ulceration**

- Venous disease 80%
- Arterial disease
- Vasculitis
- Trauma
- Burns
- Pressure sore
- Obesity
- Immobility
- Diabetes
- Peripheral neuropathy
- Cancer: basal or squamous cell cancer
- Pyoderma gangrenosum

Table 45.2 **How to use Doppler to measure Ankle Brachial Pressure Index (ABPI)**

1. Wrap blood pressure cuff around upper arm
2. Place Doppler probe over brachial artery in antecubital fossa (same site where stethoscope normally placed)
3. Inflate then slowly release pressure until Doppler detects return of pulse
4. Repeat on leg, with cuff around lower thigh and Doppler probe over artery behind medial ankle
5. If (ankle pressure)÷(arm pressure) >0.9: no arterial disease

Table 45.3 **Burns assessment**

- **Burn Area assessment**
  - assess roughly using 'Rule of Nines' (see Fig. 45.9)
  - assess more accurately using Handprint concept
  - one Handprint area = approx 1% body surface area (see Chapter 10)
- **Burn Depth assessment**
  - superficial partial — epidermis lost
  - deep partial — epidermis and dermis lost
  - full thickness — epidermis, dermis and subcutaneous fat lost

  Assess clinically 2 days after burn. If no capillary refill after pressure or stretching, suggests deep partial or full thickness

Fig. 45.1
Venous eczema with ill-defined erythema and crusting

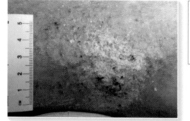

> ▶ **Warning**
>
> In venous eczema there is a risk of cellulitis or ulceration, consider pressure stockings.

Fig. 45.2 **Atrophie blanche at ankle**

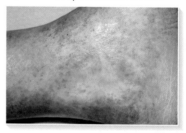

Fig. 45.3
Bilateral lipodermato-sclerosis – firm woody feel

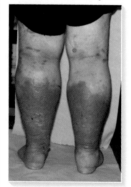

Fig. 45.4
Venous ulcer at ankle with surrounding haemosiderin

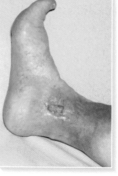

Fig. 45.5
Arterial ulcer dorsum of foot with surrounding cellulitis

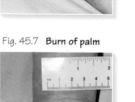

Fig. 45.9
Rule of Nines, rough percentages to assess area of burns

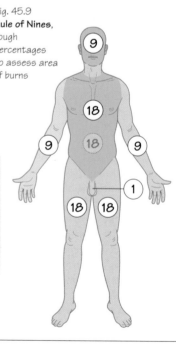

Fig. 45.6
Neurotrophic ulcer, distal sole

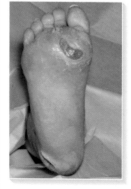

Fig. 45.7 **Burn of palm**

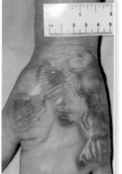

Fig. 45.8 **Burn reaction to cryotherapy**

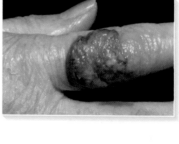

Dermatology at a Glance, First Edition. Mahbub M.U. Chowdhury, Ruwani P. Katugampola, and Andrew Y. Finlay.

Leg ulcers

An ulcer is defined as a break in the skin with loss of epidermis or also dermis. Leg ulcers have a major impact on quality of life causing social restriction and pain, costing the UK NHS £400 million each year. There are many causes of leg ulcers (Table 45.1).

Venous hypertension and pathogenesis of venous ulcers

The pressure in the veins in the lower leg depends on the height of blood directly above pressing down: this is usually 0–20 mmHg. Disease of the veins, immobility and obesity results in the valves in the large veins in the leg not working properly (incompetent) and so the pressure rises above 20 mmHg (venous hypertension). This high pressure results in leakage of fluid (oedema) and fibrin from the veins into the dermis. Fibrin cuffs form around the small veins in the dermis, causing venous insufficiency and ulceration.

Venous eczema (stasis dermatitis, gravitational eczema, varicose eczema) (Figure 45.1)

Occurs on the lower legs and is itchy. There is mild scaling with redness and oozing. The hyperpigmentation looks like melanin but is caused by dermal haemosiderin from red blood cells.

Treatment: emollients and low potency topical steroids.

Atrophie blanche

Small white atrophic lesions typically near a painful lower leg ulcer, with red dots (large capillaries) visible. May suggest other systemic inflammatory disease (e.g. SLE) (Figure 45.2).

Lipodermatosclerosis

A hard painful 'wooden feeling' area around the lower leg, with overlying redness and palpable edge (Figure 45.3). The leg shape may look like an upside down cola or wine bottle. It is caused by long-standing venous hypertension, chronic inflammation and fibrin in dermis and underlying fat. Often confused with cellulitis, but this is inflammation without infection. There is a high risk of ulceration. Compression may help long term but is 'too late'.

Examination of leg ulcers (Figure 45.4)

Ninety-five per cent of venous leg ulcers are near the ankles. Examine the nearby skin for atrophy, hair follicle loss, pitting oedema, pigmentation or sign of other disease such as malignancy.

Management of leg ulcers

Investigations
- Measure ankle brachial pressure index (ABPI) (Table 45.2).
- Check haemoglobin, white cell count or CRP (?infection), serum glucose and sickle-cell test if at risk.
- Biopsy if malignancy suspected.

Venous leg ulcer treatment: compression bandaging

Sustained compression is much more important to the outcome than the type of dressing. Only use if a Doppler study (Table 45.2) confirms no arterial disease. Evidence based benefit with optimum healing taking 4 months if compression pressure is 40 mmHg at the ankle. Use four or three layer compression bandaging and elevate the leg when sitting or lying down. Obese or oedematous ankles need more bandages to maintain pressure. Encourage weight loss and increased mobility. Maintain treatment as 25% risk of recurrence after 1 year.

Antibiotics and ulcers

All wounds have surface bacteria. Only treat pathogenic organisms if there is clinical evidence of bacteria doing harm. Give systemic antibiotics if surrounding cellulitis, redness, tenderness or exudate of pus. Avoid topical antibiotics as they encourage growth of resistant organisms, do not reach the bacteria that cause cellulitis deep within the skin and may cause contact dermatitis.

Risk of allergic contact dermatitis

Multiple topical preparations may be used for chronic ulcers. The skin barrier is already broken so it is easy for allergens to get in (e.g. antibiotics, preservatives, lanolin, rubber in elastic bandages).

How an ulcer heals

Granulation tissue forms as an early response to injury. Re-epithelialisation starts from the edge and from any persisting appendages such as hair follicles within the ulcer. Newly formed keratinocytes migrate across the wound beneath the scab.

Other ulcers (Figures 45.5 and 45.6)

Pressure sores

Normally people turn over during sleep, but they cannot turn if immobile (e.g. after a stroke). If over many days the pressure of the weight of the body goes through one area such as a bony prominence, the skin will become relatively ischaemic and may ulcerate. Pressure sores must be prevented by regular turning of immobile patients and by using special weight distributing mattresses. Pressure sores take months to heal and can be disastrous, complicating rehabilitation after illness. Bed sore frequency is an indicator of the quality of nursing care.

Arterial ulcers (Figure 45.5)

Occur on toes, feet, shins, with well-defined edges and severe pain. Most common cause atheroma: essential to stop smoking.

Treatment: if ABPI very low, surgery to restore blood flow.

Pyoderma gangrenosum

Ulcers occur at odd sites, with undermined purple edges. Associated with rheumatoid arthritis, inflammatory bowel disease, leukaemia and IgA monoclonal gammopathy. High dose systemic steroids are indicated.

Burns (Table 45.3; Figures 45.7–45.9)

Burns may be from fire, electricity or chemicals and cause permanent scarring, major disability or death. Common in mobile infants (e.g. cooker, hot water): there is a need for prevention strategies.

Emergency treatment: put out the flames (e.g. by rolling the patient in a blanket), and cool the injured site with cold water. Maintain airway and get to hospital fast.

Management: fluid replacement; careful estimation as overhydration can be dangerous. Control pain and maintain body core temperature. Consider transfer to specialised burns unit.

Long-term management: management of scarring and risk of squamous cell carcinoma in scars (Marjolin ulcers).

Key points
- Compression bandaging is critical for venous leg ulcers.
- Do not confuse lipodermatosclerosis with cellulitis.

Table 46.1

Examples of hereditary skin disease and their mode of inheritance

- **Autosomal recessive (AR):** xeroderma pigmentosa (see Chapter 40), recessive dystrophic epidermolysis bullosa
- **Autosomal dominant (AD):** ichthyosis vulgaris, Darier's disease, epidermolysis bullosa simplex, bullous ichthyosiform erythroderma, neurofibromatosis 1, tuberous sclerosis
- **X-linked recessive (XLR):** X-linked recessive ichthyosis
- **X-linked dominant (XLD):** incontinentia pigmenti

Table 46.2

What to do when a hereditary skin disease is suspected

- Detailed clinical history, including detailed family history of the suspected disease manifestations
- Thorough clinical examination of the affected individual and, when possible, other affected relatives
- Blood from index case and, when possible, relatives for DNA analysis to identify disease-causing mutation(s)
- Skin biopsies may be required for histological examination for characteristic features of the disease
- Refer patient and relatives for genetic counselling, pre-natal and/or ante-natal counselling and testing

Table 46.3 **Characteristics of some inherited ichthyoses**

Disease	Inheritance	Pathogenesis	Clinical features
Ichthyosis vulgaris (Fig. 46.1)	AD	Filaggrin	Fine scales on trunk, large scales on legs, spares flexures
X-linked recessive ichthyosis (Fig. 46.2)	XLR	Steroid sulphatase	Affects males, females are carriers. Fine to large dark scales on trunk, limbs and sides of face
Bullous ichthyosiform erythroderma (Fig. 46.3)	AD	Keratin 1 or Keratin 10	Erythroderma and blistering at birth and neonatal period followed by marked hyperkeratosis on trunk and limbs, with a velvety appearance, prominent on flexures
Netherton syndrome	AR	SPINK5	Erythroderma, double-edged scale, bamboo appearance of hair-shafts, high serum IgE
Harlequin ichthyosis	AR	ABCA12	Thick, large plates of scale encase the neonate at birth. Most die within few weeks

Table 46.4 **The main types of epidermolysis bullosa (EB)**

Disease	Inheritance	Pathogenesis	Clinical features	Level of blister formation in the skin (see Fig. 17.1)
EB simplex	AD	Abnormal keratin 5 or 14	Blistering mainly of the palms and soles	Epidermis (intraepidermal)
Junctional EB	AR	Abnormal laminin or type XVII collagen	Skin fragility with denuded skin, often on axillae and groins, may be more widespread	Lamina lucida and lamina lucida-densa interface of the basement membrane
Dystrophic EB	AD or AR	Type VII collagen	Hands and feet with marked scarring and deformities	Sublamina densa of the basement membrane

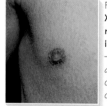

Fig. 46.1
Ichthyosis vulgaris
– note the fine scaling on the trunk

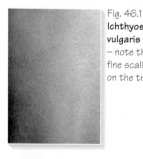

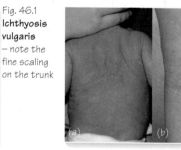

Fig. 46.3
Bullous ichthyosiform erythroderma
(a) note the generalised erythroderma and scaling of the trunk
(b) note the marked hyperkeratosis with a velvety appearance on flexures

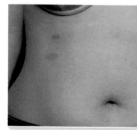

Fig. 46.6
Café-au-lait macules in NF1

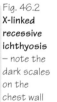

Fig. 46.2
X-linked recessive ichthyosis
– note the dark scales on the chest wall

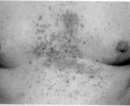

Fig. 46.4
Darier's disease of the chest wall

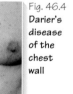

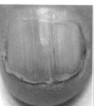

Fig. 46.5
Notching of the distal nail plate in Darier's disease

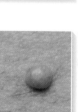

Fig. 46.7
Neurofibroma in NF1

Dermatology at a Glance, First Edition. Mahbub M.U. Chowdhury, Ruwani P. Katugampola, and Andrew Y. Finlay.

There are a vast number of hereditary skin diseases. Examples of hereditary skin diseases and the clinical approach are summarised in Tables 46.1 and 46.2.

Ichthyoses

These are a group of inherited disorders resulting in abnormal keratinisation, differentiation and desquamation of the epidermis (Table 46.3). They are characterised by generalised scaling of the skin to varying degrees from mild (ichthyosis vulgaris) to severe life-threatening (harlequin ichthyosis). Ichthyoses usually present at birth, in the neonatal period or early infancy. Presence or absence of erythroderma or blistering, distribution and features of the scale help to differentiate between the ichthyoses.

Diagnosis can often be made clinically and confirmed by the characteristic histological features on skin biopsy ± DNA analysis to identify disease causing mutation(s) ± biochemical analysis for defect in disease-causing molecules.

Treatment is symptomatic, aimed at decreasing the hyperkeratosis: topical emollients, keratolytics (10% urea or 5% salicylic acid), retinoids. Oral retinoids (acitretin) may dramatically improve some forms of ichthyosis. However, the benefits of life-long use need to be weighed against its potential side effects and use in women of child-bearing age (teratogenic).

Epidermolysis bullosa

A group of inherited disorders where different disease-causing mutations result in defects in the structural proteins of the basement membrane (see Chapter 17, Figure 17.1). Characterised by skin fragility and blistering following minor trauma, ulceration and infection of wounds followed by scarring.

Mucosal surfaces may be affected: eyes, gastrointestinal tract (e.g. dysphagia due to oesophageal strictures may lead to nutritional deficiencies and complications such as iron-deficiency anaemia).

There are three main types, with many subtypes of varying severity according to the level of blister formation in the skin (Table 46.4).

Diagnosis is made clinically and confirmed by the characteristic electron microscopic features on skin biopsy and DNA analysis.

Treatment is supportive and aimed at:
- **Avoiding or minimising skin trauma:** use of foam pads to pressure points, elbows and knees; non-adherent dressing for wounds.
- **Avoiding or managing infected wounds** with antibiotics.
- **Nutritional support:** multi-vitamin and iron supplementation.
- **Monitoring** chronic non-healing wounds for evidence of malignant transformation to squamous cell carcinoma and its prompt treatment in the dystrophic forms of epidermolysis bullosa.

Darier's disease

An autosomal dominant disease: mutations in the *ATP2A2* gene on chromosome 12 interfere with intracellular Ca^{2+} signalling. Characterised by red–brown keratotic crusted papules on the trunk and face which are often prone to secondary bacterial infection (Figure 46.4), palmar pits and notching of distal nail plate (Figure 46.5).

Treatment: antimicrobial washes, keratolytic emollients (with 10% urea), topical retinoids or corticosteroids, oral retinoids (acitretin).

Neurofibromatosis 1 (NF1)

An autosomal dominant neuro-cutaneous disease: mutations in neurofibromin gene on chromosome 17 result in loss of its tumour suppressor effect and uncontrolled cell growth.

Cutaneous manifestations: café-au-lait macules (Figure 46.6). These are light brown macules up to several centimetres in diameter that develop in childhood, ≥6 macules is one of the diagnostic features of neurofibromatosis 1. Neurofibromas are derived from peripheral nerves and their surrounding tissue (Figure 46.7). These are multiple soft pedunculated skin-coloured nodules that develop in older children and young adults. Large painful plexiform neurofibromas and axillary freckling may also develop.

Extracutaneous manifestations: ocular (Lisch nodules on iris, optic nerve glioma), neurological (involvement of the spinal cord or brain with neurofibromas), malignant change (sarcomas).

Diagnosis is made clinically; can be confirmed on DNA analysis. MRI of brain and spinal cord is required for symptomatic patients. No specific treatment is available except surgical excision of troublesome or disfiguring neurofibromas.

Tuberous sclerosis

This is an autosomal dominant neuro-cutaneous disease caused by mutations in genes encoding tumour suppressor proteins harmartin (chromosome 9) and tuberin (chromosome 16).

Cutaneous manifestations: ash-leaf macules (oval, hypopigmented macule(s) appear in infancy), adenoma sebaceum (firm, skin-coloured/erythematous papules of the face, especially on the naso-labial region appear in childhood), shagreen patches (skin-coloured patch with papular surface, usually seen on the lower back), peri-ungual fibromas (firm skin-coloured papules).

Extra-cutaneous manifestations: neurological (seizures, learning disabilities), ocular (retinal phacomas: grey–yellow plaques near the optic disc), tumours (cardiac rhabdomyomas, angiomyolipomas, astrocytomas).

Diagnosis is made clinically; can be confirmed on DNA analysis. MRI is helpful in identifying tumours. No specific treatment is available. Surgical or laser treatment can be useful for disfiguring or troublesome adenoma sebaceum and peri-ungual fibromas.

Key points

- A detailed family history is essential in inherited skin diseases.
- Genetic counselling should be offered to those with inherited skin diseases.
- The mainstay of management of ichthyosis is emollients and/or keratolytics and acitretin for severe cases.
- For epidermolysis bullosa avoid or prevent skin trauma and wound infections.
- Inherited skin diseases may be associated with extra-cutaneous complications.

▶ Warning

- Some inherited skin diseases are complicated by malignant transformation of skin or extra-cutaneous tissue.
- Oral retinoids (acitretin) can be beneficial in some inherited skin disorders. However, acitretin is teratogenic so use it with extreme caution in women of child-bearing age.

Clinical picture quiz

Answer True or False to the following questions.

Case 1

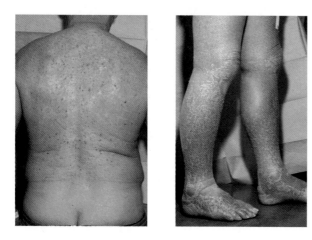

This man presented with a widespread red scaly rash affecting most of his face, body, arms and legs. He had a previous history of well-defined scaly plaques on his knees and elbows.

1 *This patient has erythroderma.*
2 *The most likely underlying cause for this patient's current skin status is psoriasis.*
3 *This patient is at risk of hyperthermia.*
4 *This patient is at risk of cardiac failure.*
5 *All patients with this skin manifestation should be treated with systemic steroids.*

Case 2

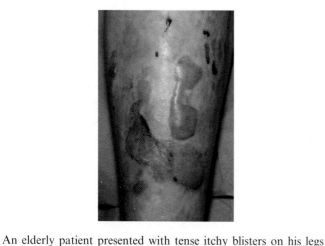

An elderly patient presented with tense itchy blisters on his legs and trunk.

1 *The most likely diagnosis is bullous pemphigoid.*
2 *The oral mucosa is never affected in this skin disease.*
3 *Direct immunofluorescence is essential to confirm the diagnosis.*
4 *This patient's skin blistering may be associated with coeliac disease.*
5 *Localised areas of this condition can be treated with topical steroids.*

Case 3

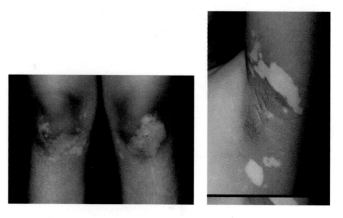

This patient presented with gradually enlarging, non-itchy, non-scaly white patches on both knees and axillae.

1 *The most likely diagnosis is vitiligo.*
2 *May be associated with thyroid disease.*
3 *Topical corticosteroids should not be used for treating this condition.*
4 *UVB or UVA phototherapy can be used to treat this condition.*
5 *Repigmentation following treatment may be patchy.*

Case 4

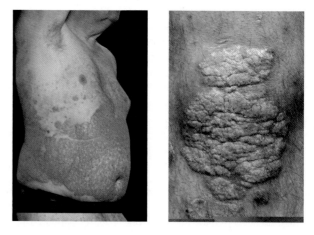

This patient presented with a several year history of thick, scaly, erythematous plaques on his trunk, elbows and knees.

1 *The most likely diagnosis is psoriasis.*
2 *This rash typically occurs in an asymmetrical distribution.*
3 *The scalp, nails and joints may be affected in this condition.*
4 *This disease does not demonstrate Koebner's phenomenon.*
5 *Widespread disease can be treated with UVB phototherapy.*

Dermatology at a Glance, First Edition. Mahbub M.U. Chowdhury, Ruwani P. Katugampola, and Andrew Y. Finlay.

Case 5

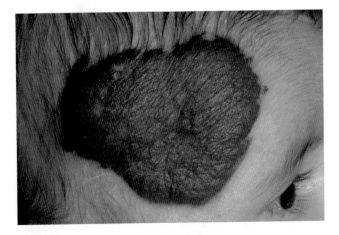

This rapidly growing red lesion appeared within the first few weeks of life of this otherwise well infant.

1 *The most likely diagnosis is a vascular malformation.*
2 *These lesions usually regress spontaneously over years.*
3 *These lesions may bleed and/or ulcerate.*
4 *These lesions should always be treated with systemic steroids.*
5 *Oral propranolol is used to treat these lesions if they interfere with function or rapidly enlarge.*

Case 6

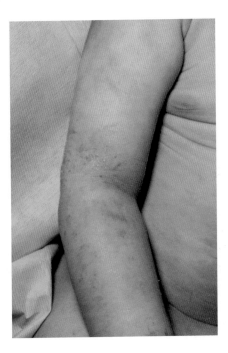

This child gave a history of an itchy dry rash since the age of 3 months. The rash affected the face, body and limbs, and was worse on the skin creases of limbs.

1 *The most likely diagnosis is atopic dermatitis.*
2 *Epidermal barrier function is usually defective in this condition.*
3 *Pitting of nails is a common finding in these patients.*
4 *This rash may be complicated by herpes simplex virus infection.*
5 *Topical corticosteroids are the treatment of choice in this condition.*

Case 7

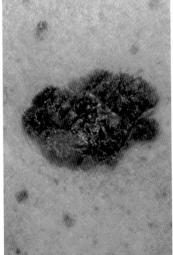

What is the diagnosis for this presentation and what other lesions could this be confused with?

1 *The incidence of this type of skin growth is reducing.*
2 *These cause 80% of skin cancer deaths.*
3 *Red hair increases the risk of developing melanoma.*
4 *Change in shape of a mole suggests possibility of melanoma.*
5 *A partial skin biopsy is ideal for diagnosis.*

Case 8

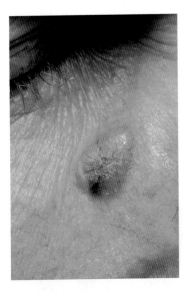

What different types of this skin cancer do you know?

1 *This the most common type of human malignancy.*
2 *These tumours are aggressive and grow rapidly.*
3 *A biopsy is always needed to confirm the diagnosis.*
4 *Mohs' surgery is indicated for treatment of ill-defined skin cancers.*
5 *These occur in sun exposed sites.*

Case 9

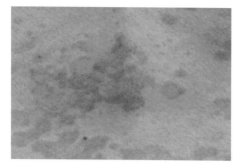

What is the diagnosis of this presentation and what history would you need to take?

1 *This condition is usually non-itchy.*
2 *The chronic form lasts more than 6 weeks.*
3 *Bizarre shapes can occur.*
4 *Angio-oedema of the face is rare.*
5 *The mainstay of treatment is anti-histamines.*

Case 10

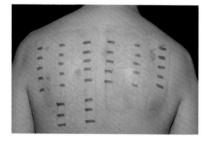
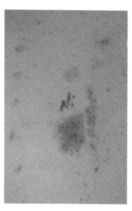

What test is shown here and what are the indications?

1 *This test detects type I allergy.*
2 *This test detects type IV allergy.*
3 *This test can diagnose irritant contact dermatitis.*
4 *Allergic contact dermatitis caused by nickel is common.*
5 *Allergic contact dermatitis can co-exist with atopic eczema.*

Case 11

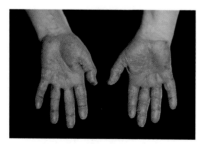
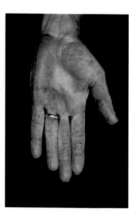

What is the most likely diagnosis for this presentation?

1 *This condition is usually itchy.*
2 *Psoriasis of the hands can be made worse with friction.*
3 *Tinea usually affects both hands.*
4 *Hairdressers are at increased risk of this condition.*
5 *Potent topical steroids are indicated.*

Case 12

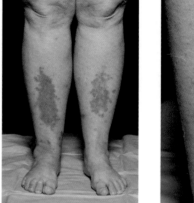
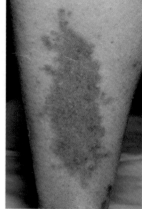

What is this condition?

1 *This occurs in diabetics.*
2 *This usually occurs on the legs.*
3 *This can be treated with topical steroids.*
4 *This can be treated with phototherapy.*
5 *This improves with better diabetic control.*

Case 13

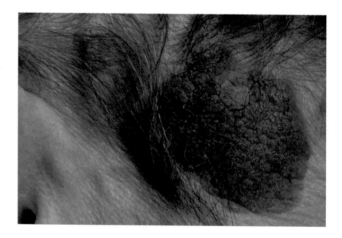

What is the most likely diagnosis for this presentation?

1 *These lesions are benign.*
2 *These commonly occur on the trunk of the elderly.*
3 *These can be of variable pigmentation.*
4 *These always need to be removed.*
5 *These have no malignant potential.*

Clinical picture quiz answers

Case 1
1 True (for further details on erythroderma see Chapter 16).
2 True. The clinical description of the patient's previous rash is suggestive of psoriasis (for further details on psoriasis see Chapter 12).
3 False. Patients with erythroderma are at risk of hypothermia.
4 True
5 False

Case 2
1 True (for further details on bullous pemphigoid see Chapter 17).
2 False
3 True (for further details on immunofluorescence see Chapter 17).
4 False. Dermatitis herpetiformis (not pemphigoid) can be associated with coeliac disease (for further details on dermatitis herpetiformis see Chapter 17).
5 True

Case 3
1 True (for further details on vitiligo see Chapter 37).
2 True
3 False
4 True
5 True

Case 4
1 True (for further details on psoriasis see Chapter 12).
2 False
3 True
4 False. Koebner's phenomenon is the appearance of skin lesions on sites of trauma, often in a linear distribution. The following skin diseases demonstrate this phenomenon: psoriasis, lichen planus, vitiligo, viral warts, molluscum contagiosum.
5 True (for further details on phototherapy see Chapter 39).

Case 5
1 False. This is an infantile haemangioma (for further details on haemangiomas and differentiating features between vascular malformation and infantile haemangiomas see Chapter 26).
2 True
3 True
4 False
5 True

Case 6
1 True (for further details on atopic dermatitis see Chapter 13).
2 True
3 False (for further details on nail pitting see Chapter 25).
4 True
5 True (for further details on topical corticosteroids see Chapter 10).

Case 7
1 False
2 True
3 True
4 True
5 False

Discussion
This is a malignant melanoma (for diagnostic criteria and types of melanoma see Chapter 35).
• Other pigmented lesions that most commonly cause confusion with malignant melanoma include moles, pigmented basal cell carcinomas and seborrhoeic keratoses.
• Malignant melanoma incidence has increased steadily over the last 40 years. A full excision with a 2-mm margin is ideal for initial diagnosis. A partial biopsy can be difficult to interpret histologically (e.g. depth: Breslow thickness) to determine prognosis.

Case 8
1 True
2 False
3 False
4 True
5 True

Discussion
This is a basal cell carcinoma (BCC) (see Chapter 34 for types of BCC).
• BCCs are slow growing and usually only locally invasive, metastasis is very rare.
• Initial clinical diagnosis can be sufficient for most BCCs with histological confirmation after removal. However, a biopsy is required if there is any doubt.
• Sun exposure is an important risk factor for BCC.

Case 9
1 False
2 True
3 True
4 False
5 True

Discussion
This is urticaria (for history points see Chapter 32 and Table 32.2).
• Urticaria is usually very itchy and this can be the main problem in some patients.
• Chronic urticaria lasts greater than 6 weeks with no cause found in 80%.
• Bizarre shapes such as annular patterns can be seen.
• Angio-oedema of the face including lips and eyelids can occur in up to 50% of patients.
• Anti-histamines are the main treatment used (see Table 32.4).

Case 10
1 False
2 True
3 False

4 True
5 True

Discussion

This shows the back on day 4 after patch testing. A nickel allergy reaction is seen (see Chapter 30).
• Patch testing is a specialized technique applying allergens to the back to detect delayed type IV hypersensitivity. This does not diagnose irritant contact dermatitis but excludes allergic contact dermatitis if negative.
• Nickel is the most common metal allergen detected. Exposure is common in many metal objects such as jewellery.
• Any patient with treatment resistant atopic or endogenous eczema should have patch testing to exclude allergic contact dermatitis.

Case 11

1 True
2 True
3 False
4 True
5 True

Discussion

This picture shows hand eczema (see Chapter 31).
• This is usually itchy and 5–10% of the population are affected during their life. Other differential diagnoses include psoriasis and tinea (see Table 31.1).
• Psoriasis can be worsened with friction and tinea manuum is usually unilateral.
• Certain occupations (e.g. hairdressing) are more prone to hand eczema including irritation and allergy.
• Potent topical steroids can be used for short periods (e.g. 6 weeks).

Case 12

1 True
2 True
3 True
4 True
5 False

Discussion

This is necrobiosis lipoidica (see Chapter 41).
• Necrobiosis lipoidica occurs in diabetics and usually affects the shins. Better diabetic control does not lead to improvement.
• Topical steroids and PUVA phototherapy can be used but both may be unsatisfactory.

Case 13

1 True
2 True
3 True
4 False
5 True

Discussion

This shows a seborrhoeic keratosis (see Chapter 33).
• Seborrhoeic keratoses are benign and very common on the trunk of elderly patients.
• Variable pigmentation of seborrhoeic keratoses can cause diagnostic confusion with malignant melanoma. However, they have no malignant potential and do not need to be removed if clinical diagnosis is confident.

Index